HUMAN HEALTH

A Bio-cultural Synthesis

The Author

Dr. Subir Biswas (b. 1974) teaches Anthropology at West Bengal State University since 2009 as a Reader. Before that he was engaged with North Bengal University since 2001 as a Lecturer. He obtained his Masters Degree in Anthropology from Calcutta University and Ph.D. from North Bengal University. In course of his association with N.B.U., he has experienced with several field works within the range of Northern part of West Bengal. His areas of interest include Anthropological Demography, Health and Bioethics. He has in his credit three research projects of University Grants Commission and Centre for Women's Studies, NBU; as well as several research articles of Anthropological interests. He has presented research papers at many conferences in India and abroad. He is a member of several professional Anthropological Associations. Email: gargisubir@gmail.com

HUMAN HEALTH

A Bio-cultural Synthesis

Subir Biswas
Reader and Head
Department of Anthropology
West Bengal State University
Barasat, Kolkata (West Bengal)

CONCEPT PUBLISHING COMPANY PVT. LTD.
NEW DELHI-110059

ISBN-13: 978-81-8069-846-0

First Published 2012

Published and Printed by

Concept Since 1974

Concept Publishing Company Pvt. Ltd.
A/15-16, Commercial Block, Mohan Garden
New Delhi-110059 (India)
T: 25351460, 25351794, *F*: 091-11-25357109
E: publishing@conceptpub.com, W: www.conceptpub.com
Editorial Office: H-13, Bali Nagar, New Delhi-110 015. India.

Cataloging in Publication Data--*Courtesy:* D.K. Agencies (P) Ltd. <docinfo@dkagencies.com>

Human health : a bio-cultural synthesis / [editor], Subir Biswas.
p. cm.
Includes bibliographical references and index.
ISBN 9788180698460

1. Public health—India—Congresses. 2. Tribes—Health and hygiene—India Congresses. 3. Tribes—Nutrition—India—Congresses. 4. Tribes—Anthropometry—India—Congresses. 5. Physical anthropology—India—Congresses. I. Biswas, Subir, 1974-

DDC 362.10954 23

Preface

World Health Organization defines Health as a state of complete physical, mental and social well-being and not merely the absence of disease or infirmity. Therefore, health includes physical, social and psychological well-being. Two models of Bio-cultural research predominate in health studies; first one integrates biological, environmental and cultural data, whereas, second one is more segmented model where biological data are primary in nature and others are secondary. Anthropologists and social scientists criticize such models when biological studies ignore the role of social, cultural or political stressors. Hence an additional dimension having more emphasis on socio-cultural aspects is also recommended.

Anthropologists, working on said aspects, are realizing that both biological and social factors need to be considered to understand human health. Anthropologists examine the major health issues that affect most human societies, describing and synthesizing the ways in which biology, culture, health, and environment interact. Therefore, the subject itself is developing as 'Bio-cultural syntheses'.

The present work is an outcome of two national seminar entitled "Human Health: A Bio-cultural Synthesis" (Phases I and II) organized by Department of Anthropology, West Bengal State University during March 2010. It intends to explore such field of Anthropology and related health sciences to understand it from the holistic point of view. Therefore, it is not only related to biological or genetic aspect of health, but also socio-cultural influences on human health.

The seminar(s) was sponsored by Anthropological Survey of India, Ministry of Culture, Government of India and Indian Council of Medical Research, Ministry of Health and Family Welfare, Govt. of

India. It was possible to organize successfully only through the active participation of students and faculty members of the Department of Anthropology, West Bengal State University. I would like to thank my colleagues Dr. Abhijit Das and Mr. Debasis Kumar Mondal for valuable help and co-operation. I am grateful to Prof. Ashoke Ranjan Thakur, the Honourable Vice-Chancellor of our University for financial support, kind permission and guidance to arrange the seminar(s). I am thankful to all the delegates from various parts of the country for their active participation. Last but not the least; I want to express my thanks to my wife, Dr. Gargi Biswas (Saha) for co-operation and support during seminar days.

Keeping in mind the importance and application of the topic, twenty one selected papers are being included in this volume.

The first article "Health and Disadvantaged People: Emerging Challenges and Opportunities" by Prof. B. Chaudhuri is a classic example of studying health in respect of bio-demographic as well as socio-cultural-economic even environmental context. The article by Dr. Chaturbhuj Sahu "Indigenous Knowledge of the Health and Disease among the Tribal Community of Hazaribagh district, India" is about traditional knowledge and practices related to health as well as recent changes with specific examples from Santhal and Birhor of said area. Dr. Jesurathnam Devarapalli in his article "Success to Human Health: Medical Monopoly or Pluralism" explains the way ethnomedicine and biomedicine go hand-in-hand to form an integrated medical system. In another article "The Challenges of Medical Pluralism: A Brief description on some basic Issues", Mr. Aritra Samajdar and Dr. Jesurathnam Devarapalli examine and explore different types of medical systems prevailing among Indian societies with examples from a village of West Bengal. Dr. Sumita Chaudhuri in her paper "Health and Urban Poor" compares and highlights on different health issues among Beggars of Kolkata after comparing data of different time period. Dr. Pranjal Boruah in his paper "Socio-Cultural Dimension of Health Care Practices: A Study among the Ao-Nagas of Nagaland" examines the differentials in health care practices among the said tribe of Nagaland with special emphasis on economy, food habit, living condition and resources. The title of the paper by Mr. Thambi Durai Thangavel and Dr. Jesurathnam Devarapalli indicates that they endeavour to point out "The Role of Food Habits and Social Practices in Understanding the Health Care of Kurichchan of Krishnagiri district of Tamil Nadu". Dr. Samar Kumar Biswas in his article "Suicide: An Anthropological

Study at Sagar Block, West Bengal" describes how natural environmental hazards affect normal life of the population which in some cases leads to suicide or attempt to suicide. Dr. Soma Bandyopadhyay in her paper "Death in Homeland is Sweeter than Life in Elsewhere to the People of Jadugoda" found health hazards because of radioactive contamination due to uranium mine of said region. Mr. Biswanath Gan in his paper "Child Worker and Its Effect on Health: A Study on Stone Crushing Sector" examines health, hygiene and medical facilities of child workers engaged in stone crushing. Dr. Suchismita Sen Chowdhury in her article "Rural Health Care System and Women Health: A Comparative Study on India and Bangladesh" describes and compares health care programmes and health care institutions/units of two neighbouring countries.

Dr. Rajesh K. Gautam, Dr. Dipak K. Adak and Prof. Premananda Bharati in their paper "Role of Climate in Anthropometric Variation: A Study among Central Indian Population" examine how climatic factor regulates variation in anthropometric characters. Dr. Jyoti Ratan Ghosh and Prof. Arup Ratan Bandyopadhyay in their article "Assessing Obesity in Adult Bengalee Males in India" have examined obesity based on different BMI cut-off values and recommend the better ones. Dr. N.K. Bagchi and Dr. D.K. Adak in their article "Metabolic Syndrome in a Peri-urban Condition: The Paundra Kshatriya of South 24 Parganas, West Bengal" describe prevalence of metabolic syndrome on said population as well as related anthropometric indicators. Dr. Shruti Agrawal and Dr. Pratiti Ghosh in their article "Food Habits and Diseases: Some Observations" deal with the food habits of Bengalee and Biharees and correlate it with genetic diseases. Dr. Ratna Bhattacharya in her paper "Nutritional Status of a Tribe: The Bharias of Patalkot" has tried to assess nutritional status of said group with special emphasis on land carrying capacity. Dr. Haradhan Mondal in his article "Reproductive Performance among the Namasudra: A Study on Location Distance" deals with various aspects of reproductive performance on different locations among said population. Dr. Amlan K. Ray, Dr. Samiran Bisai, Dr. Kaushik Bose, Dr. Shraboni Ray, Dr. M. Roy Choudhury and Dr. J. Bhattacharya in their paper "Etiological Factors, Assisted Reproduction and Pregnancy Outcome: A Retrospective Observation among Infertile Couples" correlate pregnancy outcome with the factors causing infertility as well as assisted reproduction with special emphasis on age and genital tuberculosis. Mr. Chittranjan Mondal in "Pattern of Adolescent Growth among the Bhotia Boys" describes adolescent growth pattern of the group with some comparison with neighbours. Ms. Jhillika Paul in her article "Trepanation: A Surgical Operation practiced in Prehistoric Society" has tried to document the said practices with prehistoric evidences. The last one "Automatic Testing of Colour Blindness" by Dr. Sandip Dey, Dr. Sirsendu Shekhar Ray and Dr. Kaushik Roy is description of a computerized programme to identify colour vision deficiencies.

I hope that this book would help researchers, policy-makers, administrators and workers working in the field of human health to understand the same as a bio-cultural synthesis.

Subir Biswas

Contents

Part 2

Contributors

Prof. Buddhadeb Chaudhuri, Former Dr. Ambedhar Chair Professor in Anthropology, University of Calcutta, 35, Ballygunj Circular Road, Kolkata-700019, India, E-mail: buddhadebc@gmail.com

Dr. Chaturbhuj Sahu, H.O.D. Anthropology, Vinoba Bhave University, Hazaribag, Jharkhand, India, E-mail: csahu_anthro@yahoo.com

Dr. Jesurathnam Devarapalli, Assistant Professor, Department of Anthropology, Pondicherry University, Puducherry-605014, India, E-mail: drjesudev@gmail.com

Aritra Samajdar, Research Scholar, Department of Anthropology, Pondicherry University, Puducherry-605014, India, E-mail: aritra.samajdar@gmail.com

Dr. Sumita Chaudhuri, UGC Research Scientist, Department of Anthropology, University of Calcutta, 35, Ballygunj Circular Road, Kolkata-700019, India, E-mail: sumita_chau@hotmail.com

Dr. Pranjal Boruah, Assistant Professor, Department of Anthropology, Dibru College, Dibrugarh-786003, Assam, India, E-mail: anthroboruah@yhaoo.com

Thambi Durai Thangavel, Research Scholar, Department of Anthropology, Pondicherry University, Puducherry-605014, India, E-mail: akttdrai@gmail.com

Dr. Samar Kumar Biswas, Assistant Professor, Department of Anthropology, University of North Bengal, Raja Rammohunpur, Darjeeling-734013, West Bengal, India, E-mail: smrkbis@yahoo.co.in

Dr. Soma Bandyopadhyay, Assistant Professor, Department of Anthropology, Sree Chaitanya College, Habra, North 24 Parganas, West Bengal, India, E-mail: somabanerjee_scc@yahoo.co.in

Biswanath Gan, Research Scholar, Department of Anthropology, University of North Bengal, Raja Rammohunpur, Darjeeling-734013, West Bengal, India, E-mail: biswanath_gan@rediffmail.com

Dr. Suchismita Sen Chowdhury, Research Fellow, Deptt. of Anthropology, University of Calcutta, West Bengal, India, E-mail: s_senchowdhury@yahoo.com

Dr. Rajesh K. Gautam, Assistant Professor, Department of Anthropology, Dr. H.S. Gour Central University Sagar, Madhya Pradesh-470003, India, E-mail: goutamraj@rediffmail.com

Dr. Dipak Kumar Adak, Research Associate (Physical), Anthropological Survey of India, 27, Jawaharlal Nehru Road, Kolkata-700016, India, E-mail: adakdipak@gmail.com

Prof. Premananda Bharati, Professor, Biological Anthropology Unit, Indian Statistical Institute, 203, Barrackpore Trunk Road, Kolkata-700108, West Bengal, India, E-mail: bharati@isical.ac.in

Dr. Jyoti Ratan Ghosh, Assistant Professor, Department of Anthropology, Visva Bharati, Sriniketan-731236, West Bengal, India, E-mail: jrghosh@visva-bharati.ac.in

Prof. Arup Ratan Bandyopadhyay, Professor, Department of Anthropology, University of Calcutta, 35, Ballygunj Circular Road, Kolkata-700019, India, E-mail: arbaner@rediffmail.com

Dr. N.K. Bagchi, Research Associate (Physical), Anthropological Survey of India, 27, Jawaharlal Nehru Road, Kolkata-700016, India, E-mail: niloy.bagchi@rediffmail.com

Dr. Shruti Agrawal, Lecturer, GMSM Mahavidyalaya, Bireswarpur, South 24 Parganeas, West Bengal, India. E-mail:shrutiagrawal74@yahoo.co.in

Dr. Pratiti Ghosh, Reader, Department of Physiology, West Bengal State University, Barasat, Kolkata-700126, West Bengal, India, E-mail: pratiti_ghosh@yahoo.co.in

Dr. Ratna Bhattacharya, Associate Professor and Head, Department of Anthropology, Bangabasi College, 19, Rajkumar Chakraborty Sarani, Kolkata-700 009, West Bengal, India. E-mail: dharam2004@gmail.com

Dr. Haradhan Mondal, Former Associate Professor, Department of Anthropology, Dinobandhu Mahavidyalaya, Bongaon-743235, North 24 Parganas, West Bengal, India.

Dr. Amlan K. Ray, Chief Communication Executive, Deptt. of Reproductive Medicine, A.H. IVF and Infertility Research Centre, 533, Jodhpur Park, Kolkata-700068, West Bengal, India, E-mail: humanedestiny@gmail.com

Dr. Samiran Bisai, Dr. D. S. Kothari Post-Doctoral Fellow, Department of Anthropology, North Eastern Hill University, Shilong-793022, Meghalaya, India, E-mail: samiranbisai@yahoo.com

Dr. Kaushik Bose, Associate Professor, Department of Anthropology, Vidyasagar University, Midnapore-721 102, West Bengal, India, E-mail: banda@vsnl.net

Dr. Shraboni Ray, Sr. Communication Executive, Deptt. of Reproductive Medicine, A.H. IVF and Infertility Research Centre, 533 Jodhpur Park, Kolkata-700068, West Bengal, India. E-mail: temple718@gmail.com

Dr. M. Roy Choudhury, Sr. Embryologist, Deptt. of Embryology, A.H.IVF and Infertility Research Centre, 533, Jodhpur Park, Kolkata-700068, West Bengal, India, E-mail; madhumita_mrc@yahoo.com

Dr. J. Bhattacharya, Director, A.H. IVF and Infertility Research Centre, 533, Jodhpur Park, Kolkata-700068, West Bengal, India, E-mail: joyb@vsnl.com

Chittaranjan Mandal, Research Associate (Physical), Anthropological Survey of India, 27, Jawaharlal Nehru Road, Kolkata-700016, West Bengal, India, E-mail: mandal.cr@rediffmail.com

Jhilika Paul, Research Scholar, Department of Anthropology, West Bengal State University, Barasat, Kolkata-700126, West Bengal, India, E-mail: debiph1@vsnl.net

Dr. Sandip Dey, Asst. Professor, Deptt. of IT, Camellia Institute of Technology, Madhyamgram (Badu Road), Kolkata, West Bengal 700129, India, E-mail: dishandip@gmail.com

Dr. Sirsendu Shekhar Roy, Asstt. Professor, Deptt. of Biotec and Medical Engineering, NIT Rourkela, Rourkela-769008, Orissa, India, E-mail: sirsendu.iitkgp@gmail.com

Dr. Kaushik Roy, Reader, Deptt. of Computer Science, West Bengal State University, Barasat, Kolkata-700126, West Bengal, India. E-mail: kaushik.mrg@gmail.com

PART 1

1

Health and Disadvantaged People: Emerging Challenges and Opportunities

Buddhadeb Chaudhuri

I

The World Health Organisation (WHO) defines health as "a state of complete physical, mental and social well-being and not merely the absence of disease and infirmity." It is well recognised that health is not the exclusive domain of medical science. To understand health and health related problems in a proper perspective, it is very important to consider the socio-cultural issues, economic dimensions and environmental aspects. This is more relevant in the context of tribal people particularly living in the rural areas.

Every culture, irrespective of its simplicity and complexity, has its own beliefs and practices concerning diseases. No culture works in a meaningless fashion in its treatment of diseases. Every culture evolves its own system of medicine in order to treat diseases in its own way. This treatment of disease varies from group to group.

The different tribal communities in India do not represent a homogenous group. There is considerable variation in the context of economy, lifestyle, behaviour and practices. Similarly, variations are also there in the context of demographic features. Thus, population of communities varies from around 20 as in the case of the Andamanese to over 40 lakhs as in the case of the Gonds. Thus in one context, the survival of the community may be most crucial factor while in another context economic development may be more important. If we examine the growth rate of tribal population it is obvious that the growth rate of the total tribal population is quite high and in fact it is higher than the all-India average. But it does not really reflect the true situation as considerable variation is there, so far the growth rate of the different tribal communities is concerned. In fact, it would be wrong to categorise the tribals as homogenous group, as there are tribal groups where: (1) the population is decreasing, (2) the population is stagnant, (3) the population is increasing, and (4) the population is increasing very fast. In case of some communities, there is a definite decline, threatening the survival of the community. In this context, the study of socio-cultural habits and health practices becomes imperative. The decline might not be only because of a lower rate of fertility but also owing to high mortality and problems in the existing health practices. The decline may be related to their food habits or certain types of food that the tribals consume which may adversely affect the fertility of the concerned population. Again, it may be worthwhile to examine what is the minimum viable population of a group. In other words, it may be examined, whether the size of the population is, in any way, related to decline, if so, what is the size. Unfortunately, till today we do not have many studies to answer some of these crucial questions.

In the first part of this presentation, a discussion will be made on certain health indicators and the health situation particularly focusing on the four states of eastern region while in the second part, an attempt will be made to examine the relationship of health with environment with particular reference to the tribals to identify the challenges and opportunities.

II

The National Health Policy formulated in 1983 and 2002 have yielded results but in several areas, the outcome has not been as expected.

Government initiatives in the pubic health sector have recorded some noteworthy successes over time. Smallpox and Guineaworm Disease have been eradicated from the country; Polio is on the verge of being eradicated; Leprosy, Kala Azar, and Filariasis can be expected to be eliminated in the near future. There has been a substantial drop in the Total Fertility Rate and Infant Mortality Rate. The success of the initiatives taken in the public health field is reflected in the progressive improvement of many demographic indicators over time.

Table 1.1: Achievements Through the Years: 1951-2000

Indicator	*1951*	*1981*	*2000*
Demographic Changes			
Life Expectancy	36.7	54	64.6
Crude Birth Rate	40.8	33.9	26.1
Crude Death Rate	25	12.5	8.7
IMR	146	110	70
Diseases			
Malaria (cases in million)	75	2.7	2.2
Small-Pox (No. of cases)	>44,887	Eradicated	
Guineaworm (No. of cases)		>39,792	Eradicated
Polio		29709	265

While noting that the public health initiatives over the years have contributed significantly to the improvement of these health indicators, it is to be acknowledged that public health indicators/disease-burden statistics are the outcome of several complementary initiatives under the wider umbrella of the developmental sector, covering Rural Development, Agriculture, Food Production, Sanitation, Drinking Water Supply, Education, etc. Despite the impressive public health gains as revealed in Table 1.1, one cannot deny the fact that the morbidity and mortality levels in the country are still unacceptably high. These unsatisfactory health indices are, in turn, an indication of the limited success of the public health system in meeting the preventive and curative requirements of the general population.

Out of the communicable diseases which have persisted over time, the incidence of Malaria staged resurgence in the1980s before stabilising at a fairly high prevalence level during the 1990s. Over the years, an increasing level of insecticide-resistance has developed in the malarial vectors in many parts of the country. In respect of TB, the public health scenario has not shown any significant decline in the pool of infection amongst the community, and there has been a distressing trend in the increase of drug resistance to the type of infection prevailing in the country. A new and extremely virulent communicable disease—HIV/AIDS—has emerged on the health scene since the declaration of the NHP-1983. As there is no existing therapeutic cure or vaccine for this infection, the disease constitutes a serious threat, not merely to public health but to economic development in the country. The common water-borne infections—Gastroenteritis, Cholera, and some forms of Hepatitis—continue to contribute to a high level of morbidity in the population, even though the mortality rate may have been somewhat moderated.

Life expectancy at birth has increased for male and female in India. It is 64.1 years for males and 65.8 years for females (2005). This has revealed the decrease in death rate and the better improvement of quantity and quality health services in India. However, there are inter-state, inter-district and rural-urban differences in life expectancy at birth due to low literacy, differential income levels and socio-economic conditions and beliefs. In Kerala, a person at birth is expected to live for 73 years while in states like Bihar, Assam, Madhya Pradesh, Uttar Pradesh, etc., the expectancy is in the range of 55-60 years.

The infant mortality rate has declined in India from 70 infants per 1000 live births in 1999 (SRS) to 57 in 2005-06 per 1000 live births. Under-five mortality rate per 1000 live births is 85 in 2002. According to MMR-RG, maternal mortality ratio per 1,00,000 live births is 301 in 2003.

A diverse set of factors are thought to be associated with maternal mortality: factors that influence delays in deciding to seek medical care, in reaching a place where care is available, and in receiving appropriate care. The tenth plan document of India has targeted to reduce the IMR to 45 per 1000 live births by 2007 and 28 per 1000 live births by 2012. The main causes of high MMR being socio-economic status of women, inadequate ante-natal care, the low proportion of institutional deliveries, and the non-availability of skilled birth attendants in two-thirds of cases.

A World Health Report (1999) gives the main causes of mortality in India as non-communicable diseases (48%), communicable diseases (42%) and injuries (10%). The dominant communicable diseases are infectious and parasitic diseases, respiratory diseases, maternal conditions, perinatal conditions and nutritional deficiencies. Non-communicable diseases are malignant neoplasm, diabetes mellitus, neuropsychiatric disorders, sense organ disorders, cardiovascular diseases, respiratory diseases, digestive diseases, congenital anomalies, oral diseases and other non-communicable diseases.

NFHS-II conducted a study on four major diseases prevailing in India, i.e., asthma, tuberculosis, jaundice, malaria. In India around 2,468 persons per 1,00,000 populations were reported to be suffering from asthma at the time of survey. The prevalence of asthma is high in rural areas than in urban areas and is slightly higher in males than in females. The overall prevalence of tuberculosis in India is 544 per 1,00,000 populations. This is 16 per cent higher than the survey done by NFHS-I

Table 1.2: Variations in Health Status Among States

Sector	*Population BPL (%)*	*IMR/ Per 1000 Live Births (1999-SRS)*	*<5 Mortality per 1000 (NFHS-II)*	*Weight For Age- % of Children Under 3 years (<-2SD)*	*MMR/ Lakh (Annual Report 2000)*	*Leprosy cases per 10000 population*	*Malaria +ve Cases in year 2000 (in thousands)*
India	26.1	70	94.9	47	408	3.7	2200
Rural	27.09	75	103.7	49.6	—	—	—
Urban	23.62	44	63.1	38.4	—	—	—
Better Performing States							
Kerala	12.72	14	18.8	27	87	0.9	5.1
Maharashtra	25.02	48	58.1	50	135	3.1	138
Tamil Nadu	21.12	52	63.3	37	79	4.1	56
Low Performing States							
Orissa	47.15	97	104.4	54	498	7.05	483
Bihar	42.60	63	105.1	54	707	11.83	132
Rajasthan	15.28	81	114.9	51	607	0.8	53
Uttar Pradesh	31.15	84	122.5	52	707	4.3	99
Madhya Pradesh	37.43	90	137.6	55	498	3.83	528

(467 per 1,00,000). It is more in case of rural areas than in urban areas and more for male than females. It is more in males because of males are in contact with more people who might have TB and smoking is more in men. The prevalence of TB increases with age. Jaundice cases were reported to be 1361 persons per 1,00,000 populations. This is more prevalent in rural areas than in urban areas. However, it decreases with age. Thus, highest numbers of jaundice patients are in the age group of 0-14. 3,697 persons per 1,00,000 populations were reported to have suffered from malaria. People of rural area suffer twice than that of urban area and it is slightly high for males than for females. All these diseases however vary and differ from state to state depending on the climate and geographical locations of the areas.

In the period when centralized planning was accepted as a key instrument of development in the country, the attainment of an equitable regional distribution was considered one of its major objectives. Despite this conscious focus in the development process, the facts given in Table 1.2 clearly indicate that the attainment of health indices has been very uneven across the rural-urban divide.

The statistics bring out the wide differences between the attainments of health goals in the better-performing States as compared to the low-performing States. It is clear that national averages of health indices hide wide disparities in public health facilities and health standards in different parts of the country. Given a situation in which national averages in respect of most indices are themselves at unacceptably low levels, the wide inter-State disparity implies that, for vulnerable sections of society in several States, access to public health services is nominal and health standards are grossly inadequate. Despite a thrust in the NHP-1983 and 2002 for making good the unmet needs of public health services by establishing more public health institutions at a decentralized level, a large gap in facilities still persists.

Historically, it has been the practice to implement major national disease control programmes through the public health machinery of the State/Central Governments. It has become increasingly apparent that certain components of such programmes cannot be efficiently implemented merely through government functionaries. A considerable change in the mode of implementation has come about in the last two decades, with the increasing involvement of NGOs and other institutions of civil society. It is to be recognized that widespread debate on various public health issues has, in fact, been initiated and sustained by NGOs and other members of the civil society. Also, an increasing contribution is being made by such institutions in the delivery of different components of public health services. Certain disease control programmes require close interaction with the beneficiaries for regular administration of drugs; periodic carrying out of pathological tests; dissemination of information regarding disease control and other general health information. NHP-2002 will address such issues and suggest policy instruments for the implementation of public health programmes through individuals and institutions of civil society.

Environmental and Occupational Health

The environmental conditions are a significant determinant of the health risks to which a community is exposed. Unsafe drinking water, unhygienic sanitation and air pollution significantly contribute to the burden of disease. Work conditions in several sectors of employment in the country are sub-standard. As a result, workers engaged in such employment become particularly vulnerable to occupation-linked ailments. The long-term risk of chronic morbidity is particularly marked in the case of child labour. NHP-2002 has tried to address the risk faced by this particularly vulnerable section of society.

National Rural Health Mission (NRHM) under the Ministry of Health and Family Welfare (MHFW), Government of India has recently (2008) brought out a document entitled "India Guaranteeing Quality Primary Health Care for All: An Agenda for Action". The public health challenges have been identified state-wise and are shown in Table 1.3:

Table 1.3: Health Problems in Bihar, Jharkhand, Orissa and West Bengal

Indicator	*States with High Incidence/Low Performance*
Infant Mortality	Orissa, Bihar
Maternal Mortality	Bihar, Orissa
High expenditure in Government Hospitals	Bihar, Orissa
High TB cases/suspect cases	Jharkhand, Bihar, West Bengal
High TFR	Bihar, Jharkhand
Full Immunization	Bihar, Jharkhand
Diabetes	West Bengal
Asthma	West Bengal
Malaria	West Bengal, Orissa, Jharkhand
Tobacco & Alcohol	Bihar, Jharkhand, Orissa, West Bengal
Diarrhoea & availability of ORS	Jharkhand
HIV prevalence	Nil

So it is seen that the high incidence of communicable diseases including vector-borne malaria, dengue, water-borne diarrhoea and hepatitis and air-borne pneumonia, measles, T.B. are quite common in this region. Incidentally, all these diseases are due to poverty, malnutrition and certain environmental factors like poor sanitation and unsafe drinking water. Now there is a growing trend to give more emphasis on non-communicable diseases than on communicable diseases which affect a much larger segment of the population, primarily the disadvantaged people and can be reduced, if not eliminated, if certain efforts are made and without much financial commitment.

It may not be out of context to start with population growth in the region which is given in Table 1.4.

Table 1.4: Population from 1971 to 2001 (Population figures in 000's)

State/Country	*Population*			
	1971	*1981*	*1991*	*2001*
Bihar	56353	69914	64530	82998
Jharkhand	—	—	21843	26945
Orissa	21944	26370	31659	36804
West Bengal	44312	54580	68077	80176
India	548159	683329	846421	1028737

Table 1.5: Population Distribution (in Percentage), 2001

State/Country	*Below 6 yrs*	*10-19 yrs*	*Working Age (15-59 yrs)*	*Elderly Popn. 60+yrs*
Bihar	20.2	22.0	51.1	6.6
Jharkhand	18.4	22.4	54.3	5.9
Orissa	14.6	21.1	58.4	8.8
West Bengal	14.2	21.4	59.5	7.5
India	15.9	21.9	57.1	7.3

Table 1.6: Sex Ratio (1991, 2001)

	1991	*2001*	*Absolute Change*
Bihar	907	919	+12
Jharkhand	922	941	+19
Orissa	971	972	+1
West Bengal	917	934	+17
India	927	933	+6

Table 1.7: Child Sex Ratio (1991, 2001) (Girls per 1000 boys)

	1991	*2001*	*Absolute Change*
Bihar	953	942	–11
Jharkhand	979	965	–14
Orissa	967	953	–14
West Bengal	967	960	–7
India	945	927	–18

Table 1.8: Infant Mortality Rate (IMR)

	1971	*1981*	*1991*	*2001*
Bihar	–	118	69	62
Jharkhand				
Orissa	127	135	124	91
West Bengal	–	91	71	51
India	129	110	73	66

Table 1.9: Anaemia among Children (6-59 months) and Women (15-59 yrs)

	Any Anaemia (children)	*Any Anaemia (women)*
Bihar	78.0	67.4
Jharkhand	70.3	69.5
Orissa	65.0	61.2
West Bengal	61.0	63.2
India	69.5	55.3

The above demographic features show a number of disturbing trends. The sex ratio is not very encouraging; in Bihar, it is much below the national average and in the best performing state, Orissa, the improvement is not much. But the most disturbing feature is the child sex ratio which shows a gradual decline at the national level and all the four states under consideration. It speaks of a demographic imbalance in future. Even though there is some improvement in the context of infant mortality rate in all the states of this region, still it is quite high. Again, the prevalence of anaemia is quite conspicuous in the context of all states in this region both for the children and women.

III

Access to, and benefits from, the public health system have been very uneven between the better-endowed and the more vulnerable sections of society. This is particularly true for women, children and the socially disadvantaged sections of society. The facts given in Table 1.10 highlight the handicap suffered in the health sector on account of socio-economic inequity.

Table 1.10: Variations in Health Status among Socio-economic Groups

Indicator	*Infant Mortality/1000*	*Under 5 Mortality/1000*	*% Children Underweight*
India	70	94.9	47
Social Inequity			
Scheduled Castes	83	119.3	53.5
Scheduled Tribes	84.2	126.6	55.9
Other Disadvantaged	76	103.1	47.3
Others	61.8	82.6	41.1

So it is seen that child mortality including under five child mortality and underweight children are more found among the Scheduled Tribes, then Scheduled Caste and other disadvantaged groups. Considering these negative health indicators, it is obvious that these communities need special attention.

Science in Society: Indigenous Wisdom and Knowledge

Despite our entire technological breakthrough, we still live in a world where a fifth of the developing world's population goes hungry every night, a quarter lacks access to even basic necessity like safe drinking water and a third lives in a state of object poverty—at such a margin of human existence that words simply fail to describe it. In both developing and industrial countries, the threats to health security are usually greater for the poorest, people in the rural areas particularly the indigenous people. Spending on health programmes is also very different and it is quite low in the developing countries; for example it is only $7 per individual per year in Bangladesh. Considering this alarming situation, out of the seven important targets put forward for human development in the Agenda for Social Summit, four were related to health. They are as follows:

- Primary health cares for all with special stress on the immunization of children.
- Severe malnutrition to be eliminated and moderate malnutrition rates to be halved.

- Family planning services for all willing couples.
- Safe drinking and sanitation for all.

The prevailing health and medical system, the western system, has unfortunately failed to meet the need of the world's majority. The failure of the *Alma Ata* Declaration in fulfilling its objectives of achieving Health for All by the year 2000 gives more urgency for looking for an alternative. In most countries a very frightening policy change is being manoeuvred by agencies like the World Bank and IMF (International Monetary Fund) to give less and less emphasis to the social and welfare sectors and higher emphasis to the economic and infrastructure sectors. As such the financial allocation for health is going down in most Asian countries. The implication of such a trend in countries where health insurance is unaffordable to the majority is unimaginable. Based on current trends in health care financing and the failure of the *Alma Ata* Declaration to take a grip of the situation there is an imperative need for evolving an alternative. In this whole changing situation, the condition of the poor, particularly the indigenous people has become more critical and difficult.

Generally, when we talk or think about science, we refer to the western or industrial society. In the context of scientific development, we prefer to discuss more about the so-called modern scientific innovations assuming that science is only there in those societies and quite often implying that scientific rigour or interest is absent in other societies. The role of science is to help mankind to meet the various demands exploiting the natural resources in the best possible way without adversely affecting the environment. People have developed their own science and technologies based on the demands of the concerned societies, but quite often these are ignored. What I want to impress here is that we need to look at indigenous science and technology particularly when an exiting body of knowledge is available: perhaps it is better to develop it instead of replacing it in the name of scientific development and modernization.

Health and Culture

The belief in the interference of supernatural agency is particularly strong in the case of their main economic pursuits and in the context of health and disease. The different economic activities are associated with rituals. Similarly, different deities and spirits are connected with various types of diseases. Most of their socio-cultural activities revolve around Gods and spirits. Thus, they have specific Gods for their health and disease, for calamities, for the cattle and so on.

It is important to understand and identify the cause of illness as the nature of treatment is intimately connected with it. The present author has noted this link in his study of the Mundas; Valunjkar and Chaturvedi (1967) too have noted this relationship. Religious performances occupy a prominent place in the treatment of disease, like small-pox and plague which are associated with supernatural causes. Lewis (1958) too had noted that the advantage in learning about the indigenous beliefs and practices of the community is the insight that give into the worldview of the people as concepts of disease causation are part of a society's total worldview, which is also reflected in other spheres such as agriculture, politics and interpersonal relations.

Health, Medicine and Community

Health and treatment reflect the social solidarity of a community. In a tribal community, for example, illness and the consequent treatment is not always an individual or familial affair, but the decision about the nature of treatment is taken at the community level. In the rural areas, in case of some specific diseases, not only the diseased person or his/her family, but the total village community is affected. All the other families in the village are expected to be observed certain taboos or norms and food habits. The non-observance of such practices often calls for action by the village council. One cannot deny the impact of this psychological support in the context of treatment and cure.

In most of the tribal communities, there are number of folklores related to health. Certain practices are suggested to avoid illness or diseases, while some are prescribed to have better health. These should not be ignored as mere folk-beliefs, but need careful attention. There are different folklores to avoid illness, during illness, regarding food and so on. Documentation of such folklores available in different socio-cultural system may be very rewarding and may provide the model for appropriate health practices in a given eco-system.

Medicine Men and Community

Among the tribals, there are a group of specialists—the priests and/or magicians or medicine men whose services are sought after, depending on the cause of the illness. The dependence on and confidence in traditional medicine men or magicians and shamans are again often responsible for the non-acceptance of modern medicine. The traditional approach establishes faith and assurance in the patients, while modern medicine lacks this. As the shamans or what are called traditional medicine men and magicians share the common cultural beliefs and practices of the patients, naturally they have more faith in them. Carstairs (1955), a medical psychiatrist and anthropologist, pointed out that the difference between the points of view of the physician and the village folk with regard to theories of etiology, techniques of curing and conceptions of roles of the physician, resulted in misunderstandings between himself, a physician, and his clients. Marriott (1955) has shown how the contrasts and conflicts between the roles assumed by the indigenous and the western medical practitioners resulted in obstacles to the acceptability of western medicine.

Health, Food Habits and Nutrition

It has been noted by many that tribals living in remote areas have a better health status and more balanced food than those living in less remote areas (Chaudhuri, 1986; Chaudhuri *et al.,* 1989). In two projects related to tribal health, it has been noted that the various roots and tubers available in the forest or small animals they can hunt supply a more balanced nutritional status of the tribals as most of the roots and tubers are not available (Chaudhuri:2003). Again, in many cases, it has been noted that certain diseases may be common in certain areas but they remain controlled because of certain food habits based on vegetation available locally or certain practices which have been generated through tradition. There is no doubt that any disturbance in the ecosystem is likely to affect the balance and adversely affect the concerned population.

Another survey has shown that contrary to the general expectation, the shifting cultivating tribes like the Padam, Riang were having better nutritional status than those of the settled agricultural tribes like the Santal and the Ho. Again, in the context of deforestation, the hunting and gathering tribes were having lower nutritional status. It is quite significant that death rates are consistently lower than the national average in some of the tribal predominant states. Roy Burman (1990) has noted that physical well-being of the tribals is inextricably linked up with the forest ecology. In fact rapid disappearance of forest, commercialisation of minor forest produce, replacement of food crops by cash crops and tendency towards monoculture forestry and lastly privatization of communal lands may affect the health and nutrition and physical well-being of the tribal population.

Health and Forest

The relation of forest with nutrition may be mentioned. It has been noted by many that the tribals living in remote areas have a better health status and more balanced food than those living in less remote areas. The various roots and tubers available in the forest or small animals they can hunt supply a balanced nutrition to hem. There is no doubt that deforestation is likely to affect the nutritional status of the tribals as most of the roots and tubers are not available. Again, in many cases, it has been noted that certain diseases may be common in certain areas but they are controlled because of certain food habits based on vegetation available locally, or certain practices which have been generated through tradition. There is no doubt that any disturbance in the ecosystem is likely to affect the balance and same diseases may spread very quickly. The mode of utilization of available natural resources often determines the long-term impact on health. A number of scholars have pointed out the nature of health hazards in the context of unplanned/ uncontrolled use of insecticides and pesticides for agricultural development. It has also been observed how this may affect the nutritional status of people, particularly the tribals. The use of insecticides and pesticides has killed the small fishes in the paddy field and thus the poorer families, who generally consumed this protein, were deprived of it. This is also true in case of many tribal areas. Thus the whole development strategy needs critical analysis as it may adversely affect the environment and consequently the health status of the people, particularly the tribals.

Forest happens to be the main source of getting medicinal plants and animals. Naturally the different Forest Acts restricting the use and exploitation of forest resources are adversely affecting the health and treatment in tribal societies. Thus, though apparently there does not exist any relation between the forest and health of an individual, in reality, the Forest Acts; deforestation and certain types of afforestation programmes may adversely affect the health of the tribals. In some of our studies on the health care system in the tribal areas, we observed how the tribal medicine men were facing difficulties in getting medical plants. Most of the traditional medicine men, who came from the three states of Jharkhand, Orissa and West Bengal, while discussing the problems they faced in practicing their profession, all clearly pointed out the difficulties they were facing in gathering medicinal plants mainly from the forest. The success of their approach has to be analysed in this context, even if their treatment is not successful in one context.

The relation of treatment and nutrition with forest among the rural population, particularly among the tribal communities is quite obvious. The traditional herbal treatment is rather a people's knowledge and an oral tradition. In many cases, many persons in the concerned community have the knowledge and in some cases, a few selected persons, the traditional medicine men are more knowledgeable. But in any case, people depend on nature, particularly on forest for these medicinal plants. Thus deforestation and commercial afforestation of mono-plant forest (?) may seriously affect the availability of these medicinal plants. Even the nutrition may be similarly affected. Access to forest resources can affect treatment and nutrition. Some of the major problems the tribal communities are facing in general and the traditional medicine men in particular in this context are as follows:

- Deforestation and non-availability of medicinal plants and animals.
- Commercial afforestation and more emphasis on commercially important plants—consequently non-availability of herbs.
- Forest Laws and Acts restricting the use and exploitation of forest resources.
- Non-availability of medicinal plants because of commercial interest in many areas.

In the past, this knowledge base was oral and almost always transmitted verbally from one generation to another. Such knowledge is in fact still used today in many areas allover the world in the day-to-day living of many indigenous people. In several parts of Asia, apart from the folk traditions there is also a parallel classical tradition of knowledge. These classical knowledge systems have very sophisticated theoretical foundations and are codified and documented in thousand of manuscripts. They represent non-western knowledge systems of the world and very different in their worldview, concepts and principles from the western knowledge systems. Traditional knowledge in medicine and health has been time tested over generations. It is a holistic concept covering a broad base from disease prevention, health promotion and healing. It has and can deal with health problems ranging from the common cold, air and water borne diseases to orthopaedics and other complicated cases.

This system is also based on a wide range of biological resources using thousands of plant species, hundred of animal species, and animal parts and various minerals and metal sources. Unfortunately, over the years traditional knowledge and skills have been neglected and a prejudice has been engineered and encouraged by powerful nations, multinationals in order to subjugate non-western cultures.

Opportunities and Challenges

A number of myths have been systematically created against the non-western system in general and indigenous system in particular.

Often it is said that health is the exclusive domain of medical science. By restricting it in this way, the socio-economic, cultural and environmental issues are often ignored.

Following the above logic, more and more expenditure on sophisticated research is promoted. It is not my intention to discourage research but when the resources are limited, it is to be seen how best possible way the resources can be utilized and whether it should provide more expensive sophisticated facilities to a few or minimum less expensive facilities to a larger population. Perhaps there is a need to make a balance between the two.

Quite often it is said that the rural people, particularly the tribals are all superstitious. Thus if a tribal worship a deity for cure, automatically it is assumed that they are superstitious and would not accept the so-called modern health practices, but when the same thing is done in the cities of India it becomes tradition and when it is done in the Churches of Europe, it is levelled as convention. The question of rationality cannot be judged or examined in isolation, without examining the ecosystem, health facilities available and economic condition. Again, the mere presence of a health centre does not necessarily mean that people would depend on it, if proper and adequate facilities are not available or if the people are not convinced about its efficiency. In fact, bulk of the social scientists, who have studied health culture or the rural population in India have been overenthusiastic in discussing superstitious health beliefs and practices and that they have not paid adequate attention to the force which have been instrumental in causing decay and degeneration of their health culture.

The advocacy of traditional method of treatment does not mean that something counter to development is suggested. The point is that there may be many positive aspects in a traditional system, which should be encouraged and propagated. In fact, the need is to provide all the alternatives and not to depend on only one system.

The argument often put forward in favour of the introduction of the modern system (and of the replacement of the traditional) is that tribal and similar traditional approaches do not have an answer to many diseases. This is an undeniable fact but does not necessarily reflect a limitation of the traditional system. Apart from the fact of the non-availability of many herbs, one should add that many of these diseases were formerly unknown. Naturally, the question of any traditional system having a remedy for them does not arise. In fact, for the same reason, modern medicine also does not have remedies for many diseases.

Documentation of traditional knowledge in health and medicine is urgently necessary. Most of the research and publications available in this field is purely academic in nature. Society in general is schooled into thinking that adopting traditional health skill and culture is inferior as compared to modern medicine. This attitude has contributed to the further degeneration of this knowledge. Documentation is also urgently needed because the traditional knowledge is mostly an oral tradition and hence documentation is necessary before they are forgotten. Loss of this rich and diverse ecosystem based knowledge systems and skills will be no ordinary loss.

Documentation should be made and at the same time one has to be aware of the risks involved and the use the commercial interest can put to it. Hence, it should be done with certain reservations. Cases are not lacking, when after the publication of research reports on traditional medicinal plants used by the tribals, many such plants were collected in bulk by outside big industries for commercial use for profit. As a result, they are no more available to the traditional medicine men to whom they are so essential for treatment. As a result, the tribals are deprived of their traditional system without the modern system becoming accessible to them.

A knowledge and documentation of traditional tribal medicine are also urgently necessary. It is important for the modern system to begin with the base existing in the tribal society and build on it, rather than replace it. In order to achieve this, information about tribal medicinal practices should be documented before they are forgotten. A study of indigenous method of treatment may help to identify new methods of treatment of various diseases with certain modifications. In fact, a number of ethno botanical studies have helped to identify a number of medicinal plants used by the tribals to treat different types of diseases. Many of them may be very useful to treat diseases and it is urgently necessary to document them and try them after proper scientific experiment. This has been observed in the few studies that have been made on tribal medicine, especially in terms of efficiency, which is very encouraging. This, however, needs to be further substantiated by sustained research. It may be said that the achievement of tribal medicine is quite revealing. However, to utilize the research findings for further development and application for benefiting the vast majority of the rural poor, particularly the tribals who are living in areas which have very little or no so-called modern medical facilities, needs an integrated and multidisciplinary research and follow-up dissemination efforts.

Legal and policy issues involving protection of traditional knowledge also needs to be examined. A legislative framework is required whereby the knowledge is kept with the people and recognition, financial or otherwise, is accorded to the individual or community by commercial firms who have to use their knowledge.

The changing forest policies and the changing development scenario in Asian countries has adversely affected the strength of the biological resources used in traditional medicine as much of these resources are being depleted through deforestation. The mono-plant afforestation programmes where emphasis is given on commercial plants has not helped the people much. There is a need to promote conservation measures for saving medicinal plants on various eco-systems and habitat.

A number of studies have pointed out the nature of health hazards in the context of unplanned/uncontrolled use of insecticides and pesticides. It has been noted how they have killed the small fishes in the paddy field and thus the poorer families, who generally consumed this protein were deprived of it. This is also true in case of many tribal areas. Thus the whole development strategy needs critical analysis as it may adversely affect the environment and consequently the health status of the people, particularly the tribals.

Multinational drug companies, medical lobby and the western media have played a major role in disrupting and negating the indigenous knowledge systems while on the other hand exploited this traditional knowledge and resource base to develop new drugs. Current efforts at research in ethnic pharmacology have often proved to be counter-productive to the development or advancement of local cultures as the objective is not to strengthen the traditional knowledge and resource base but to get information for multinational drug companies. It is well-known that drug multinationals have been robbing traditional knowledge for their own interests.

There is a need to perpetuate and revive the traditional/indigenous system, which is close to the people, non-commercial in nature and curative in approach. It this context, it may be necessary for:

(a) identification of factors responsible for erosion of indigenous health care system and formulation of action programmes to countermand it,
(b) formulation of appropriate methodology to institute traditional health care system in rural/tribal areas, and
(c) identification of methodology for more intensive and integrated documentation, research and development.

References

Banerjee, D. 1986, *Social Science and Health Service Development in India*, Lok Paksh, New Delhi.

Chaudhuri, Buddhadeb, 1979, *Cultural Dimensions of Health: A Study on West Bengal Villages*' 1st International Congress on Traditional Asian Medicine, Canberra, Australia.

—— 1986, *Tribal Health: Socio-Cultural Dimensions*, Inter-India Publications, New Delhi.

—— 1986, Social and Cultural Aspects of Health, *Journal of Social and Economic Studies* (n.s.) 379-388.

—— 1989, 'Social Science, Health and Culture: The Tribal Situation', *Social Action*. 39(3): 243-253.

—— 1990, The Case of Tribal Medicine, in *The Philosophy of Science*, (ed.) J.V. Narlikar and others, Indian Institute of Advanced Study, Shimla.

—— 1990, *Cultural and Environmental Dimensions on Health*, Inter-India Publications, New Delhi.

—— 1993, Health, Culture and Environment: The Tribal Situation in India, in *Continuity and Change in Tribal Society*, (ed.) Mrinal Miri, Indian Institute of Advanced Study, Shimla.

—— 2003, *Forest, Health and Development: The Tribal Situation*, Inter-India Publications, New Delhi.

Chaudhuri, Buddhadeb, D. Dasgupta and K.K. Chatterjee (eds.). 1989, *Tribal Medicine*, Regional Research and Study Centre, Midnapore.

Lewis, Oscar, 1958, *Village Life in Northern India*, Random House, New York.

Jain, S.K., 1968, *Medicinal Plants*, National Book Trust, New Delhi.

Joseph, A.N.T., 1992, Ethnozoology of Reptiles in Relation to Health care among Tribals in Madhya Pradesh, in *National Development and Tribal Deprivation*, (ed.) Walter Fernandes, Indian Social Institute, New Delhi.

Marriott Mckim, 1955, Western Medicine in a Village of Northern India, in *Health, Culture and Community*, B.D. Paul (ed.) Russel Sage, New York.

Roy Burman, B.K. 1990, Development Hazards to Health in Tribal India. in *Cultural and Environmental Dimensions on Health*, (ed.) Buddhadeb Chaudhuri. Inter-India Publications, New Delhi.

2

Indigenous Knowledge of the Health and Disease among the Tribal Community of Hazaribagh District, India

Chaturbhuj Sahu

Introduction

India is famous for having second largest concentration of tribal people in the world. They are having some special salient features which make them unique. Since hoary past, these groups of people in spite of many adverse situations and confrontations here and there are in a position to sustain their tribal virility, cultural identity and indigenous knowledge of healing diseases.

The tribal people are scattered throughout the country. They are mostly inhabited in the tracts of hills and forest of sub-Himalayas, and in the eastern regions, in mountain belt of central India between Narmada and Godawari rivers and in the southern most part of the Western Ghats up to Kanyakumari. The socio-cultural and economic conditions of these tribals vary considerably and it is an accepted fact that tribal people in general are lagging far behind the population of the other sectors in every field. Vidyarthi and Rai (1977) have categorized them into eight different types from hunting gathering to skilled workers on the basis of their economic condition, but they possess knowledge of health, disease and treatment. They have their own concept of good health. They explain that health is the most valuable thing on this earth. They clearly identify about the good health and bad health. A man who is free from disease possesses good health. In this healthy situation he looks energetic and feels fit in performing his daily work smoothly and comfortably. Healthy man is regarded as an asset for family, society and nation. Health in broad sense is quality of life rather than only the absence of disease. Thus health is the primary factor and foundation stone of human personality. But in the present context health status of the tribals are not satisfied.

Hassan (1964) has observed that health and diseases are related to sociological and cultural resources of a community in a specific environment.

The health of an individual is dependent on hereditary and the environmental factors. It requires continuous adjustment to the environment as living organisms are dependent upon the environment in which they live (Kumari and Kumari 1998).

The World Health Organization defines health as "a state of complete physical, mental and social well-being and not merely the absence of disease or infirmity (cited in Lewis 1976)". The basic concept of health and disease, in this sense, needs an empirical investigation in various societies for acquiring specific details. Health and diseases are measures of the effectiveness with which a human group has adopted to the environment.

The health of any community, particularly of a tribal community by and large is a function of the interaction between the socio-cultural and socio-biological particles, the genetic attributes and the environmental conditions. The widely varying prevalent health practices are use of indigenous herbal drugs. Taboos and superstition are also responsible for determining the health behaviour and health status of the tribal groups (Sahu 1998).

Keeping all these, attempts have been made to elaborate the indigenous knowledge of health and diseases of the tribal community of study area. This knowledge has been transmitted to the next generation since their appearance on the earth as a settled life. Each generation made significant additions to this knowledge in a context adjustment to changing circumstances and environmental condition. With the passage of time this knowledge was preserved in oral traditions in modern scientific knowledge this is known as ethno-medicine.

Indigenous knowledge is not a system which has constructed at the modern knowledge producing centres like universities, laboratories and research institutes rather it was in formally constructed, deconstructed and modify in the field situation on the basis of day-to-day experiences, needs and requirement of its users. It has become user in every sphere of life including health and disease. This is equally true for the tribals of Hazaribagh district. They have their own concept of good health. They can easily diagnose about different kinds of health and diseases. They also know about the cause of disease and method of curing diseases. They have plenty of knowledge about tribal medicine used for either common disease or chronic disease and children diseases and so on.

Study Area: Hazaribagh District

Situated on the 24°59'30" latitudes and 85°22' longitudes respectively and rich in flora and fauna, Hazaribagh is a natural museum of rocks and topological inequalities. It is the headquarters of North Chotanagpur Commissionary and the Hazaribagh district. It is a region of plateaus, residual hills and valleys. It is surrounded by seven hills and hillocks namely Sitagarha, Babhanbay, Silwar, Kanhari, Vanadag, Musna and Belian. The climate of the area is very pleasant (Sahu 2001).

Hazaribagh is one of the famous districts of tribal Jharkhand. It is the home of socially and culturally impotent tribes viz. Santhal, Munda, Karmali, Badiya, Mahli and Birhor. The Oraons and Kharwars are also seen in a limited pocket.

For the present study the Santhal and Birhor tribes have taken into consideration.

Santhal and Birhor

The Santhal is one of the oldest and largest tribes of India numbering more than 4 million souls. They are found in Jharkhand, Bihar, West Bengal, Orissa, Assam and in the vicinity of India such as Bangladesh. They claim their origin in Harappa and Mohenjodro i.e. in hihri-pipiri. They, being the ancient most aboriginals of India consist a rich culture with well defined social system and life structure.

The Birhor is a vanishing, nomadic, hunters, gatherers, ropemakers, isolators and a group of half fed and half naked people. They are found in hilly areas of Jharkhand, Chhattisgarh, Orissa and West Bengal, but their main domain is Jharkhand. Their socio-economic and religious life is greatly influenced by Nature-Man-Spirit Complex (Vidyarthi 1963, Sahu 1982, 1995). Their entire life revolves round the forest.

The Birhors' great specialization is indigenous herbal medicines and in locality they are considered to be the most efficient herbal doctor. They are in great demand not only by the other tribal communities but also by many other non-tribals even.

Health Care Strategy

Though the meaning of 'health' varies from person to person, every known human society looks after the health situation of its members in different possible ways. As a result, various methods were emerged even among the tribals to cope with the health problems and to check the death rate as much as possible. The charter of the WHO founded in 1948 has mentioned that the objective of these programmes is to bring down the mortality and morbidity, physical, mental and social. But the success of any health care programme much depends on the organizations and scope of its administrative structure and the consciousness of the target group.

The National Health Policy, approved by the Parliament in 1983, is mainly concerned with the primary health care to all. The principal areas of this health care strategy are:

1. Nutrition for all.
2. Immunization.
3. Maternal and child health care.
4. Presentation of food adulteration.
5. Water supply and sanitation.
6. Environmental protection.
7. School health programme.
8. Occupational health services.
9. Prevention and control of endemic diseases.

In every health care strategy balance between women and other is necessary for tribal as well as non-tribal community.

Concept of Health among the Tribal Groups

Health is not simply just a disease free state but in holistic sense, it envisages physical, mental and social well-being of the individuals. The concept of well-being varies between different groups, yet in an environment of tribal habitat, a person is usually considered to be afflicted with some disease if he/she is incapable of doing the routine work which is usually being expected to be carried out by that individual in the society (Kshatriya 2001).

Most of tribal societies have definite means for the identifying and classifying various kinds of ailments and diseases.

There is strong belief among the tribal groups that the ancestral spirits play important role in the prosperity and protection of the family. These spirits are believed to bring a state of physical, mental and social well-being to the members of the family. In case of any trouble first of all they concern traditional diviners for appearing, controlling or driving away the disease causing agents. They remain conscious about the malevolent spirits as serious harm in the sphere of their health life.

Tribal Health Status

There is no doubt that the health status of the tribal people throughout the country is very poor. Among them varying health practices are widely prevalent like, indigenous traditional medicines, taboos and superstition. These practices are also responsible for determining the health seeking behaviour on health status i.e., fertility, mortality and morbidity patterns. Different studies (Basu 1986, 1990, Rizvi 1986, Mukherjee 1986, Swain *et al.*, 1990, Sahu 1982, 1995, 2005) have tried to establish this with the help of morbidity, mortality and health statistics. Worst status is seen among the children. They try to prevent and protect their babies with the help of indigenous medicine. In acute situation some well to do family used to come to the hospital for taking proper treatment of specialized doctors. However, their attitude towards modern medicine care is not encouraging.

Indigenous Medical System

The indigenous medical system among the Santhal and Birhor can be divided into two groups:

1. The ritual
2. The herbal medicine

The ritual medicinal system is based on enchanting of ***mantras*** by ritual specialist. The second category of medicine men are the herbal doctors who do not enchant ***mantras***, though they believe in magical action of the herbals, they use. They do not take much care about their health. They follow the traditional treatment. They feel that their disease or ill health is their physical disability. They pray to their deities for curing the diseases. They have a great faith that these diseases cannot be cured by medicines. Herbal medicine is very much prevalent among them, they consult the ***ojhamati*** for herbal medicines and spiritual cure.

The suffering of the people under study is related to the following diseases—cough, cold, fracture, vomiting, dysentery, joint pain, female disease, asthma, eye and ear trouble, fever including malaria, breathing trouble, heart disease, skin disease, acid gas, liver trouble etc. For the treatment of such diseases they perform some magico-religious performance or use herbal medicines.

The incidence and prevalence of chronic as well as non-chronic diseases are high among the aged. Some people are suffering from many diseases for a duration of more than three years. 4 per cent of them have availed the services of private and government hospital for the treatment of their ailments. Sex and age differentials among the patients of chronic diseases have been seen. Asthma is the most prevalent chronic disease among the men whereas rheumatic pains are more common among females. 60 per cent of the total (400) aged people have been suffering from various kinds of chronic ailment and acute diseases. They are in the opinion "when we are suffering from any disease we receive not satisfactory treatment". It is seen that the females are worst sufferer than the males. This is possible due to nutrition deficiency, negligence of women in the society and their low access to health care service delivery. The women are also sufferer of seasonal diseases. For healing of the seasonal diseases they use herbal medicine available in their locality. They use to take herbal medicine for the well-being and to remain free from the acute health problems. The people of study area are significantly different from other communities in case of T.B. and diabetes as not a single person has been seen suffering from these diseases.

From Table 2.1 it has been observed that there is difference between Santhal and Birhor tribe regarding treatment of the disease. 55.4 per cent Santhal male undertake indigenous treatment of the disease; while it is 93 per cent in case of Birhor tribe. Regarding Santhal women 68.3 per cent believe in indigenous treatment including ***Jharphuk*** while almost the same situation has been seen for Birhor women. 100 per cent Birhor women has not taken advantage of other methods of treatment. 77 per cent of Santhal widow's diseases are cured by

Table 2.1: Curing of disease by Indigenous/Biomedicine/Both

Tribe	*Indigenous Treatment*		*Biomedicine*		*Both*		*Total*
	No.	*%*	*No.*	*%*	*No.*	*%*	
Male Santhal	144	55.4	26	10.0	90	34.6	260
Male Birhor	40	93.0	–	–	03	7.0	43
Female Santhal	82	68.3	16	13.3	22	18.3	120
Female Birhor	25	92.6	–	–	2	7.3	27
Widow Santhal	86	77.0	06	5.8	18	17.4	104
Widow Birhor	06	100.00	–	–			06

indigenous treatment whereas only 5.8 per cent referring belief on medical treatment. 34.6 per cent Santhal males have believed in both treatments together. It is clear that Santhal is becoming conscious for taking advantage of allopathic treatment. It also indicates that there is a lack of the way of proper treatment hence an attempt needs to be made to make the people more and more conscious about it.

Table 2.2: Patients Admitted in Hospital (or not) during Last Three Years

Tribe	*Admitted*		*Not Admitted*		*Total*
	No.	*%*	*No.*	*%*	
Male Santhal	40	34.48	76	65.52	116
Male Birhor	02	14.3	12	85.7	14
Female Santhal	14	36.48	24	63.52	38
Female Birhor	–	–	04	100.0	04
Widow Santhal	08	33.33	16	66.66	24
Widow Birhor	–	–	02	100.0	02

It is found from Table 2.2 that during last three years there is no difference among the Santhal Male, Female and Widow patients admitted in hospital or any other nourishing home for curing the diseases, whereas 14.3 per cent male Birhor admitted in Sadar Hospital with the pressure of Government administration. It has been reported that in worst cases the Santhal prefer to admit the patient in hospital.

Tribal Health Care Programme

It has been seen that the country is characterized by having significant achievement in the production of drugs, pharmaceuticals vaccine, hospital equipments and other facilities for human being but sad plight to note that no special programmes of Tribal Health was introduced till the Sixth Plan period. National Health Policy, 1983 is proved the land mark for attraction of the planners in the field of Tribal Health. Hence a line of thinking began to appear during the Seventh Plan period. But actual step had been taken from 8th Plan period. In this period a Primary Health Centre was established in tribal area to cover a population of 20,000 as against in 30,000 in other areas similarly, a sub-centre was set up for a population of 3,000 in tribal areas, as against 5,000 in other areas, further relaxation was given where a habitation is more than 5 km from the nearest delivery point (Prasad and Sahu 2009).

Health Care Utilization Scheme

The utilization of modern health care facility by the tribals is non-satisfactory. It has been seen that most of the primary health centres and sub-centres are situated away from the tribal village. It takes whole day to receive the health facility centre from this centre. The health workers do not take proper interest to solve the health problems in all villages under their jurisdiction.

Some health workers want to make regular visit in their area. But the situation is not favourable for them, as they live in interior, remote and hilly areas. The doctors are also not available in their respective places. They are not taking interest to serve this needy poor tribal people.

The Santhals and Birhors are expert in collection of herbal plants which they transact with the agent of private Ayurveda Pharmaceuticals companies for meagre amount. Before deforestation it was easy to collect the herbal plants but now it has become very difficult to collect these plants. They have to move long distance with empty stomach which also affects the health status.

It has also been seen that their faith in the traditional herbs are also greater than that of any amount of modern medicines will prove useless for them. Their indigenous medicines are very rich in birth control.

Conclusion and Suggestions

The entire lifecycle of tribal communities of the study area is related to the forest. They have adjusted their routine according to the pattern of forest ecosystem. In the changing situation of the forest, they are not getting everything from the forest which is creating adverse situation for maintaining a balanced health.

Health is a basic requirement, not only for the fulfilment of human aspirations, but also for the enjoyment of all mankind of better quality of life. It is also indispensable for a balanced development of the individual within the family and as a part of the community and the nation. It also provides the ground for examining relationship between biological and social phenomenon.

The health care system among the Santhal and Birhor has not reached up to the mark due to lack of structurally modified medical and health condition. The worst situation has been seen among the Birhor. The health care system needs to be enriched by using simple, inexpensive methods and remedies derived from traditional system.

No doubt from Seventh Five Year Plan emphasis has been given towards delivering of health care and family welfare service to the rural community in general and tribal community in particular, but there is a need for popular understanding of the different health aspects of the Santhal and Birhor tribes. The widely varying prevalent health practices, use of indigenous herbal medicines, taboos and superstitions are also responsible for determining the health behaviour of them which should also be taken into consideration while making improvement programme.

Both tribes have strong faith in their own believes, customs, rituals, patterns of behaviour and ways of doing things. Many health problems are deeply rooted in their myths, taboos, and beliefs. In this context applied and action work approach is very useful for them.

Increasing number of health care facilities and technical manpower is not going to solve the health problem so the attention should be taken forward understanding their indigenous knowledge of health, felt needs and acceptance of the modern facilities.

Group discussion should be organized on the basis of their indigenous knowledge and cultural values so that they may be educated on health care.

Since most of them are quite ignorant of the proper ways and means to maintain good health and nutrition, it has been extremely difficult to achieve good health for such people. In view of the need of these people some effective and efficient ways and means should be developed to educate them, change their attitudes, and modify their practices so that they may be in a position to keep them healthy.

It is also suggested that the proposal to promote co-operation between biomedicine and indigenous medicine will be of great help and advantage to develop collaborative health care programmes.

The research should be mission oriented and directed towards improvement of the quality of life of Santhal and Birhor in particular and other tribals in general.

References

Basu, S.K., 1986. Genetics, Socio-cultural and Health Care among Tribal Groups of Jagdalpur and Kanta Tehsils of Bastar District, M.P., *In* A.K. Kalla and K.S. Singh (eds.) *Anthropology, Development and Nation Building*, New Delhi, Concept Publications.

—— 1990. *Health Scenario and Health Problems of the Tribal Population in India,* Paper presented at the Seminar on Community and Change in Tribal Society, at I.T. A.S. Shimla, Jan. 14-18.

Hassan, K.A., 1964. *The Cultural Frontiers of Health in Village India,* Bombay, Manaktalas.

Kshatriya, G., 2001. Tribal Health: Few Considerations, *In* Ramesh Chaubey and K.K.N. Sharma (eds.) *Tribal Health*, New Delhi: Inter-India Pub.

Kumari Parnita and S. Kumari, 1998. Cultural and Environmental Aspects of Health in the Santhal Tribe, *In* Chaturbhuj Sahu (eds.) *Tribal Culture and Identity*, New Delhi: Sarup & Sons.

Mukherjee, D.P. and S.K. Nandi, 1986. Anthropology of Tribal Health: A Case of the Asur in Natherhart Plateau, *In* B. Chaudhuri (ed.) *Tribal Health: Socio-cultural Dimensions*, New Delhi: Inter-India Pub.

Prasad, N. and C. Sahu, 2009. Tribal Health Development, *In* Chaturbhuj Sahu (ed.) *Approaches of Tribal Development*, New Delhi: Adhyayan Pub.

Rizvi, S.N.H., 1986. Health Practices of Jaunsaries: A Socio-cultural Analysis, *In* B. Chaudhuri (ed.) *Tribal Health: Socio-cultural Dimensions*, New Delhi: Inter-India Pub.

Sahu, Chaturbhuj, 1982. *Development of Birhor Clusters*, Ph.D. Dissertation, Ranchi University.

—— 1995. Food and Health Condition of the Birhor: A Vanishing Tribe of Bihar, *Indian Anthropologist*, 25(2): 13-24.

—— 1996. *The Santhal Women: A Social Profile*, New Delhi: Sarup & Sons.

—— (ed.), 1998. *Tribal Culture and Identity*, New Delhi: Sarup & Sons.

—— (ed.), 2001. *Indian Tribal Life*, New Delhi: Sarup & Sons.

—— (ed.), 2005. *Aspects of Tribal Studies*, New Delhi: Sarup & Sons.

Swain, S. and S.C. Jena, 1990. Morbidity Status of the Kondha Tribe of Phulbani, Orissa, *In* B. Chaudhuri (ed.) *Cultural and Environmental Dimensions on Health*, New Delhi: Inter-India Pub.

Vidyarthi, L.P., 1963. Social Anthropological Researches in India: Some Preliminary Observation, *Jr. of Social Research*, IX (1): 1-13.

Vidyarthi, L.P. and B.K. Rai, 1977. *The Tribal Culture of India*, New Delhi, Concept Publications.

3

Success to Human Health: Medical Monopoly or Pluralism

Jesurathnam Devarapalli

Introduction

Health an exclusive prerogative of medical sciences has been drawing the attention of a number of disciplines including social sciences from time to time. In fact the history of medical sciences clearly shows that it has obtained much benefit from non-medical disciplines for the status it enjoys today. This is all because of the strong relationship between health and social situations (Rosen 1963, Dubos 1965, Veith 1966). Though modern medical science is preoccupied with investigation, diagnosis and the line of treatment, the socio-economic and cultural implications of health cannot be ruled out. Hence a close coordination is needed between medical expertise and social scientists to mitigate the impasse and the role of anthropological knowledge is valuable as proposed by Galdston (1963). A number of accounts were cited by Caudill (1953) where anthropological interventions were applied to solve health and disease related problems.

Medical systems and social systems are very closely interlinked so that the advancement of one directly focuses the growth of the other. Thus, anthropological knowledge of health is understood from the two focal areas as ethnomedicine and biomedicine as pointed out by Fabrega (1972).

Ethnomedicine

It is the embodiment of cultural construct of health, disease, diagnosis and the related therapies. Owing to its culture specific theorization the universal range of application may not be possible for simple reason that what is considered the line of treatment in one culture need not be the same in another culture. However, ethnomedical practices considered in a particular society show wide ranging categories confirming pluralism in diagnosis and treatment (Devarapalli 2007).

Therapy in ethnomedicine is a vast subject that includes both magico-religious, mechanical and chemical procedures (Lieban 1973). The ethnomedical practices are based on religion, magic, massage and administering of plant and animal products externally or internally. It is not a rule that all these practices be present in all the cultures and if present, in the same frame. The indigenous medical systems appear to vary in the extent to which they depend on magic and religion (*Ibid*). A relative minimization of magic in the pragmatic orientation of Eskimo-Aleut culture was observed by Laughlin (1963) and yet in many cultures medical practices and religious practices are often fused (Glick 1967). According to Trawick (1992) in Indian thought, religion and medicine are not separate. Dodds (1959) was of the opinion that the principle of modern physiotherapy has been rooted in the ideas of massage frequently practiced by the tribes which is intended to drive away the evil spirits from the body. The use of various herbs for curing disease is nothing new in indigenous medical practices (Messing 1968, Lieban 1967).

Medical Pluralism

Modern medicine have the advantage of widely accepted theory with proven results when applied anywhere in the world. But there are a number of streams within it in the varying degree of publicity and acceptability. Thus, we see multiple systems such as Allopathy, Homeopathy, Ayurveda, Acupuncture, Unani etc. each with its own uniqueness and contradiction to the other. The idea of medical pluralism makes more sense when an individual has access to more than one cultural approach to sickness and healing and each approach need not constitute an organized system…(Press 1980).

Biomedicine

Referring to its characters the medicine is identified through a number of terms such as cosmopolitan medicine, scientific medicine, western medicine, allopathy etc. In spite of so many age old traditions thriving in different parts of the world, allopathy has excelled to its glorious heights and is ruling the arena of medical world. This is all due to its scientific temperament and great strides it has made in research creating wonders. Today we see transplantation and grafting of a number of body parts starting from the least bothered hair to the most coveted heart which are no less than marvels of allopathy that ever the world witnessed. The quick relief, often time bound, is a great boon which has taken it to all corners of the world (though it is yet to percolate into some sections of simple societies). The system is so meticulous that they put in service a number of sophisticated techniques and technologies in the process of diagnosis and treatment. The system has also excelled in its potential to predict and prevent disease.

With all its wonder working abilities, allopathy has not only mustered people's confidence *en masse* but has also effectively relegated other streams of medical systems to mere existence. In spite of its astounding performance and success allopathy has its own limitations which are of real concern. The most undesired impact is side effects. Most of the procedures of investigations (especially involving nuclear radiation), medication and tranquilization (anaesthesia) in spite of taking utmost care leaves behind mark of deleterious effects which may be of short or long-term consequences and this will be beyond proportions when life saving drugs are administered. Buying health through this system is very expensive and time consuming (getting appointment with the specialized expert) which vast majority of Indian population can ill afford (even in rich countries medical bill is a great concern). That is the reason why most of them are not able to continue the treatment as long as he/she is advised leading to aggravation and drug immunity. There are socio-psychological implications in this line of treatment where the patient in many situations is physically separated from the social environment. Exposure to so many sophisticated investigations and equipment before diagnosis really pulls down the courage of the person whosoever it is and it really disturbs his physical activity and social composure. At this juncture the idea of alternative medicine comes. Knowing pretty well the limitation of allopathy, the other streams of medicines such as homeopathy, ayurveda, unani etc. can act as complementary wherever possibility arise and feasibility exists as every medical system has its constraints.

Medical Ethnocentrism

Every medical system undermines the merit of the other, at least the practitioner in a bid to promote his professional and personal interest disregard to patients' socio-economic and disease conditions. Like ethnomedicine, biomedicine also operates within a cultural framework of values and premises (Hahn and Kleinman 1983) whereby it is no less immune to ethnocentric attitudes and fails to appreciate the excellence of the other due to the lack of scientific ground. On the contrary, the highly evolved scientific allopathy, no doubt with its high degree of success, yet has umpteen numbers of inexplicable failures while the lesser scientific systems (Homeopathy, Ayurveda etc.) have to their credit many success stories. Both these situations can be recollected by individual experiences. A meningitis case declared fatal was revived to a hopeful allopathic treatment through six hours Homeopathy drugs administration. The cases of sinusitis, piles, fistula, and fissures have a safe and permanent remedy at a thrown away cost in Homeopathy. Similarly, Ayurveda provides effective and result oriented solution to a number of neurological ailments including some kinds of paralysis through its means of massage, fomentation, *vasthi* etc. In spite of these glaring results it is difficult to advice the patients to seek these remedies for those proven cases keeping in mind the problems of side effect, better chance of recovery and cost-effectiveness due to professional bias. To cite an example of medical ethnocentrism, the House of Commons, Science and Technology Committee, London challenged the government to withdraw NHS funding from homeopathic treatment as it is "nothing more than water" for most scientists. However, Princes Foundation for Integrated Health countered it, but about 200 clinical trials fail to show homeopathic remedies work and its working construed no better than placebo. But Edward Ernst, Professor of Complementary Medicine at the University of Exeter argues; why not give homeopathic placebos if they help patients? (Boseley 2010).

Integrated Medical System

When human welfare is the primary goal of any medical system the narrow feelings of professional rivalry and ethnocentric leanings should not come in the path of any kind of alignment and aggregation. This could be possible only when there is attitudinal change among the diverse medical practitioners, by having a primary exposure to the merits of each stream. It may bring in greater advantage if the diverse medical systems play complementary role rather than exercise over monopoly. At this juncture the emerging field of euthanasia which envisages medical help to end life as the ultimate remedy for certain disease is most agonizing for any rational thinking. Sir Terry Pratchett, author of the bestselling Discworld fantasy novels advocating the euthanasia tribunals to legalize assisted death, is a cause of introspection to all systems of medicine (Kennedy 2010).

A popular adage says 'knowledge knows no boundaries'. There should be a platform of knowledge sharing whereby the different streams can share their expertise and develop a module for healthy diagnosis and treatment. The medical practitioners should have such a broad mind to appreciate, critically the achievements of others. Furthermore, accepting that every medical system operating within certain limits and inherent ills, the doctor should give truthful consultancy such that the patient can get the best and the safest possible treatment.

Conclusion

When health is the most precious treasure of life, people protect and procure it by all means which of late is increasingly culture neutral. This is to say that health catering systems and their machinery developing a culture of their own with diversities. The medical systems are meant for ensuring human welfare by providing health care facilities. In order to ensure this goal an integrated approach could be adapted such that the patient get best of the treatment which is less harmful, assure perfect remedy and monetarily affordable. When euthanasia is prescribed by the most dominating medical systems as the ultimate remedy for certain ailments that in itself defeat the scientific temperament. It is therefore indeed mandatory to search for better solutions with integrated effort as no single system is panacea for all ailments.

References

Boseley, S., 2010. Homeopathy: Snipping Between Devotees and Deniers Becomes a Full-scale Battle. *The Hindu* (Chennai Edition 24.02.2010) Cf. Guardian Newspaper 2010.

Caudill, W., 1953. Applied Anthropology in Medicine. *In* A.L. Kroeber (ed.) *Anthropology Today*, Chicago: University of Chicago Press, 771-806.

Devarapalli, J., 2007. Ethnomedical Practices of Chenchu: A Case of Integrated System. *J. Human Ecology* 22 (1): 27-33.

Dodds, J.W., 1959. The Humanist Looks at the Doctor. *In* Iago Galdston (ed.) *Medicine and Anthropology*, New York: International Universities Press.

Dubos, R., 1965. *Man Adapting*, New Haven: Yale University Press.

Fabrega, H., Jr., 1972. Medical Anthropology, *In* B.J. Siegel (ed.) *Biennial Review of Anthropology,* Stanford: University Press.

Galdston, I., 1963. Retrospect and Prospect, *In* I. Galdston (ed.) *Man's Images of Medicine and Anthropology*, New York: International Universities Press, 521-525.

Glick, L.B., 1967. Medicine as an Ethnographic Category: The Gimi of the New Guinea Highlands, *Ethnology* 6: 31-56.

Hahn, R.A. and A. Kleinman, 1983. Biomedical Practices and Anthropological Theory: Frameworks and Directions, *Annual Review of Anthropology* 12: 305-333.

Kennedy, M., 2010. Are Euthanasia Tribunals the Answer? *The Hindu* (Chennai Edition, 14th February). Cf. Guardian News and Media 2010.

Laughlin, W.S., 1963. Primitive Theory of Medicine: Empirical knowledge *In* I. Galdston (ed.) *Man's Image in Medicine and Anthropology*, New York: International Universities Press.

Lieban, R.W., 1967. *Cebuano Sorcery*, Berkely: University of California Press.

—— 1973. Medical Anthropology. *In* J.J. Honigmann (ed.) *Handbook of Social and Cultural Anthropology*, Chicago: Rand Mcnally & Co.

Messing, S.D., 1968. Interdigitation of Mystical and Physical Healing in Ethiopia, *Behaviour Science Notes* 3: 87-104.

Press, W.L., 1980. Toward a Theory of Practice, *In* Elizabeth M. Eddy and William L. Partridge (eds.) *Applied Anthropology in America*, New York: Columbia University Press, 211-233.

Rosen, G., 1963. The Evolution of Social Medicine. *In* H.E. Freeman, S. Levine and L.G. Reeder (eds.) *Handbook of Medical Sociology*, Englewood Cliffs: N.J. Prentice-Hall.

Trawick, M., 1992. Death and Nurturance in Indian System of Healing. *In* Charles Leslie and Allan Young (eds.) *Paths to Asian Medical Knowledge*, Berkely: University of California Press.

Veith, I., 1966. *The Yellow Emperors Classic of Internal Medicine*, Berkeley: University of California Press.

4

The Challenges of Medical Pluralism: A Brief Description on Some Basic Issues

Aritra Samajdar and *Jesurathnam Devarapalli*

Introduction

In responding to disease and illness, all human societies create medical systems of one sort or another. According to Charles Leslie (1980), the idea of "medical systems" is a product of ordering and systematization integral to modernization and the emergence of scientific medicine. Medical systems are social and cultural. In contrast to health systems, their boundaries are not those of biological populations, species and ecological networks, but of political organization and cultural exchange.

All medical systems consist of beliefs and practices that are consciously directed at promoting health and alleviating disease. Medicine in simple pre-industrial societies is not clearly differentiated from other social institutions such as religion and politics. Even though physicians in industrial societies often purport to practice a form of medicine distinct from religion and politics, in reality their endeavours are intricately intertwined with these spheres of social life (Barber *et al.*, 2003).

As noted by Foster and Anderson (1978), every medical system embraces a disease theory system and a health care system. The disease theory system includes conceptions of health and the causes of disease or illness. The health care systems refer to the social relationships that revolve around the healer and his or her patient. In the case of complex societies the whole system may work in an elaborate bureaucratic structure.

Regardless of their degree of complexity, all health care systems are based upon the dyadic core, consisting of a healer and a patient. The healer's role may be occupied by a generalist such as the Shaman in pre-industrial societies or the family physician in modern societies. It may also be occupied by various specialists.

In contrast to simple pre-industrial societies, which tend to exhibit a more-or-less coherent medical system, state societies manifest the coexistence of an array of medical systems, or a pattern of medical pluralism. From this perspective, the medical system of a society consists of the totality of medical subsystems that coexist in a cooperative or competitive relationship with one another (Sargent and Johnson 1996).

Types of Medical Systems

Various Medical Anthropologists have created typologies that recognize the phenomenon of medical pluralism in complex societies. Based upon their geographic and cultural settings, Dunn (1976) delineated three types of medical systems:(1) local medical systems, (2) regional medical systems, and (3) the cosmopolitan medical systems.

Local medical systems are folk or indigenous medical systems of small scale foraging, horticultural or pastoral societies, or peasant communities in state societies. Regional medical systems are systems distributed over a relatively large area. Examples of regional medical systems include Ayurvedic medicine and Unani medicine in South Asia and traditional Chinese medicine. Cosmopolitan medicine refers to the global medical system or what commonly has been called scientific medicine, biomedicine, modern medicine or Western medicine. Complex societies generally contain all three of these medical systems. India for example, has numerous local medical systems associated with its many ethnic groups.

Patterns of medical pluralism tend to reflect hierarchical relations in the larger society. Patterns of hierarchy may be based upon class, caste, racial, ethnic, regional, religious, and gender distinctions. Medical pluralism flourishes in all class divided societies and tends to mirror the wider sphere of class and social relationships. It is perhaps more accurate to say that national medical systems in the modern or post-modern world tend to be plural, rather than pluralistic, in that biomedicine enjoys a dominant status over heterodox and ethnomedical practices. In reality plural medical systems may be described as dominative medical system; one system attempts to exert, with the support of social elites, dominance over other medical systems; people are quite capable of the dual use of distinct medical systems.

In attempting to distinguish the Western medical system that became globally dominant during the previous century from alternative systems, social scientists have employed a variety of descriptive levels, including regular medicine, allopathic medicine, scientific medicine, modern medicine, and cosmopolitan medicine. Most medical anthropologists have come to refer to this form of medicine as "biomedicine".

Biomedicine has fostered a process that many social scientists refer to as medicalization. This process entails the absorption of ever-widening social arenas and behaviours into the jurisdiction of biomedical treatment.

Some Concepts

Medicalization

Medicalization also known as pathologization, is the process by which human conditions and problems come to be defined and treated as medical conditions and problems, and thus come under the authority of doctors and other health professionals to study diagnose, prevent or treat. The process of medicalization can be driven by new evidence or theories about conditions, or by developments in social attitudes or economic considerations, or by the development of new purported treatments. Medicalization is often claimed to bring benefits, but also costs, which may not always be clear. In some cases it may be negatively referred to as disease mongering. Medicalization is studied in terms of the role and power of professions, patients and corporations, and also for its implications for ordinary people whose self-identity and life-decisions may depend on the prevailing concepts of health and illness. Once a condition is classed as medical, a medical model of disability tends to be used rather than a social model (Peterson and Bunton 1997).

Biomedicine

Biomedicine, also known as theoretical medicine, is a term that comprises the knowledge and research which is more or less in common to the fields of human medicine, veterinary medicine, deontology and fundamental biosciences such as biochemistry, chemistry, biology, histology, genetics, embryology, anatomy, physiology, pathology, biomedical engineering, zoology, botany and microbiology.

Biomedicine is usually not concerned with the practice of medicine as much as it is with the theory, knowledge, and research of it; its results render possible new drugs and a deeper, molecular understanding of the mechanisms underlying disease, and thus lays the foundations of all medical application, diagnosis and treatment (Peterson and Bunton 1996).

Medical Pluralism

What has been termed a theoretical perspective on medicine as a social institution involves the use of an explanatory frame of reference for comparing sickness and healing. Of necessity, then, it involves comparisons of whole societies, and this runs into the problem of the diversity of ways of thinking and acting with respect to the medical realm that exists in societies that differ in terms of social and cultural complexity.

Consider that member of a small scale society can explain illness in terms of several different causes by means of which he or she could make sense of the illness and seek to heal it. Insofar as each orientation is different in terms of content and required practices, is even this type of simple society "pluralistic" with respect to the medical? While any of a member of "pluralistic" interpretations is possible, together, presumably, they form a coherent part of the one cultural reality of medicine of the society. In other words, all members of the society share in this cultural reality and see alternative causal explanations as that part of their one coherent picture of medicine.

An idea of medical pluralism makes more sense when an individual has access to more than one cultural approach to sickness and healing. Each approach need not constitute an organized system, leaving aside for the moment the problem of how one is to conceptualize what exactly is an "organized system" pertaining to sickness and healing (Press, 1980). Suffice it to say that when individuals are able to distinguish between more or less separate ways of explaining and handling the medical ways that differ in terms of basic propositions, explanatory mechanisms, procedures, and personnel, one can begin to speak more comfortably of medical pluralism (Peterson and Bunton 1996).

Argument

In this chapter the main argument centred with the relationship between biomedicine, medicalization and medical pluralism. Here we want to argue that medicalization of biomedicine is fully ethnocentric. Medical hegemony of biomedical system is deeply rooted with colonialism. All ancient civilizations have distinct medical systems, like Ayurveda in India. But with the progress of colonialism all systems collapsed. But which we cannot find in the centre that must left some footprints in periphery. And the main duty of an anthropologist is to find out those footprints from the periphery.

So, we cannot make any argument on the basis of that like Ayurveda as a national medical system. In the era of globalization in each and every part of the world national medical system is the biomedical system. But we can also find other type of medical systems still exists in the ways of life of every culture even in the West.

Chrisman and Kleinman (1986) developed a widely used model that recognizes three overlapping sectors in health care systems. The popular sector consists of health care conducted by sick person themselves, their families, social networks and communities. The folk sector encompasses healers of various sorts who function informally and often on a quasi-legal or sometimes given local laws or illegal basis. The professional sector encompasses the practitioners and bureaucracies of both biomedicine and professionalized heterodox medical systems. In all these sectors of medical systems we can find lot of evidence of medical pluralism over medical hegemony especially on the first two sectors.

So here to stand the hypothesis that medical pluralism is still an important issue to discuss, a good deal of importance is given to the available literature. We here mostly depend upon content analysis method. Only some basic questions were asked to 115 rural individuals through interviewing and canvassing a simple structured schedule. We also relied upon secondary source in arriving at conclusions.

To reach at the conclusions we have done some fieldwork also. Our field is a village, namely Sahanui and it is in Burdwan district of West Bengal. The village is multicaste, multi-ethnic and multi-religious. There are 240 households in the village. Out of those 240 households, 87 households are Santals. And out of that 87 households, the members of 36 households are converted into Christianity. Remaining 153 households are Hindu.

All of our 115 informants are Hindu by religion. Out of our 115 informants, 92 are male and only 23 are female. Below, we show caste-wise distribution of our 115 informants.

Caste and Gender-wise Distribution of Respondents

Caste	*Male*	*Female*
Brahmin	40	10
Kayastha	10	2
Sadgop	20	5
Tanti	1	—
Teli	1	—
Muchi	5	—
Banik	1	—
Bagdi	1	1
Bauri	10	4
Kush Khatriya	1	—
Baisya Kapali	1	1
Trishul	1	—
Total	92	23

Analysis

Ayurvedic medical system is one of the most influential medical systems in pre-colonial India. It exists till now. Until now in states like Kerala it is popular. In some parts and sections of our Bengali society now Ayurvedic medicine become fashion. Like Unani medical system among Muslims, Ayurvedic medical system is a dominant medical system among the Hindus. But British state opposes Ayurvedic medical system on the ground that it is one of the superstitious beliefs of the Hindus and as a medical system it is non-scientific. As the British state declared it illegal and did not sponsor it, so its growth becomes collapsed (Panikkar, 1992). After Independence it has come again into the scenario. But the previous century already create a big knowledge gap. Today Ayurveda exists but maximum up to the ointment for skin disease or headache or pain-relief.

So the first question posed to the respondent is do you believe in Ayurveda as a medical system. Out of 115 informants 95 give positive answer. Among them 76 are male and 19 are female. In this case we do not find any significant variation of response between upper caste and lower caste. Table 4.1 support our point.

Table 4.1: Belief in Ayurveda as a Medical System

Caste	Male		Female	
	Yes	No	Yes	No
Brahmin	31	9	7	3
Kayastha	9	1	2	—
Sadgop	16	4	4	1
Tanti	1	—	—	—
Teli	—	1	—	—
Muchi	4	1	—	—
Banik	1	—	—	—
Bagdi	1	—	1	—
Bauri	10	—	4	—
Kush Khatriya	1	—	—	—
Baisya Kapali	—	—	1	—
Trishul	1	—	—	—
Total	76	16	19	4

But when the next question arises regarding practicing Ayurveda in time of illness the number of positive answer giver fall down significantly to 42. Out of which 37 are male and 5 are female. Here we can find a marked variation of opinion on the basis of caste. The entire Ayurveda medicine taker in time of illness is coming from "Varna-Hindu" caste. We can find a similar trend in case of female also. Table 4.2 show the point.

Table 4.2: Practicing Ayurveda in Time of Illness

Caste	Male		Female	
	Yes	No	Yes	No
Brahmin	23	17	4	6
Kayastha	4	6	—	2
Sadgop	8	12	1	4
Tanti	—	1	—	—
Teli	—	1	—	—
Muchi	1	4	—	—
Banik	—	1	—	—
Bagdi	—	1	—	1
Bauri	1	9	—	4
Kush Khatriya	—	1	—	—
Baisya Kapali	—	1	—	1
Trishul	—	1	—	—
Total	37	55	5	18

And those who use it do not use it in time of what we understand by "illness". They use it only in case of minor health problems. Ayurveda used in case of pain, skin disease and headache. Somebody also use it as hair oil, hair colour and tooth paste. So using Chrisman and Kleinman (1983) model we can easily say that now Ayurvedic medical system fall under the popular sector where health care conducted by sick persons themselves or maximum their families.

The third question is regarding belief in Homeopathy as a medical system. Now, 66 males and 17 females or total of 83 out of 115 gave positive answer. Table 4.3 show this point.

Table 4.3: Belief in Homeopathy as a Medical System

Caste	*Male*		*Female*	
	Yes	*No*	*Yes*	*No*
Brahmin	29	11	9	1
Kayastha	7	3	2	
Sadgop	14	6	3	2
Tanti	1	—	—	—
Teli	1	—	—	—
Muchi	—	1	—	—
Banik	—	1	—	—
Bagdi	—	1	—	1
Bauri	7	3	2	2
Kush Khatriya	1	—	—	—
Baisya Kapali	1	—	1	—
Trishul	1	—	—	—
Total	**66**	**26**	**17**	**6**

And those 83 who believe Homeopathy practice when it comes to utility in time of illness, the number goes to 68. People also use homeopathic medicine in time of more serious illness than Ayurvedic medicine. These 68 respondents, who use homeopathic medicine in time of illness, use it in case of fever, cough, gastric problem, pain relief, dysentery, dehydration etc. And out of those 68 the majority of 56 are male and 12 are female. Table 4.4 show this point.

And the final question raised is do the respondents really think that alternative medical system is really alternative to biomedical system, shockingly 98 informants replied in negative. They cannot imagine a world without biomedical system. If the situation rose like that, about their opinion it is then hard to live. Chrisman and Kleinman (1983)

Table 4.4: Practicing Homeopathy in Time of Illness

Caste	*Male*		*Female*	
	Yes	*No*	*Yes*	*No*
Brahmin	26	14	8	2
Kayastha	6	4	1	1
Sadgop	12	8	2	3
Tanti	1	—	—	—
Teli	1	—	—	—
Muchi	3	2	—	—
Banik	—	1	—	—
Bagdi	—	1	—	1
Bauri	6	4	1	3
Kush Khatriya	1	—	—	1
Baisya Kapali	—	1	—	—
Trishul	—	1	—	—
Total	**56**	**36**	**12**	**11**

model we can also apply for Homeopathic medicine. Homeopathic medicine also falls under the self-administered medicine category. This medical system also fall under the popular sector where health care conducted by sick person themselves or maximum their families. Table 4.5 show this point.

Table 4.5: Thinking Alternative Medical System as a Real Alternative to Biomedical System

Caste	*Male*		*Female*	
	Yes	*No*	*Yes*	*No*
Brahmin	10	30	1	9
Kayastha	2	8		2
Sadgop	2	18	1	4
Tanti	—	1	—	—
Teli	—	1	—	—
Muchi	—	1	—	—
Banik	—	5	—	—
Bagdi	—	1	—	1
Bauri	—	10	1	3
Kush Khatriya	—	1	—	1
Baisya Kapali	—	1	—	—
Trishul	—	1	—	—
Total	**14**	**78**	**3**	**20**

The important observation is that people are quite capable of the dual use of distinct medical systems. Based upon her research among the Manus in the Admiralty Islands of Melanesia, Lola-Romanucci Ross (1977) identified a "hierarchy of resort" in which many people utilize self-administered folk remedies or consult folk healers before visiting a biomedical clinic or hospital for their ailments.

Same thing we can see here. Many of the informants in case of jaundice disease at first go to the village medicine man. There they take *mala*. After that they consult allopathic doctor and also take biomedicine.

Conclusion

So until now a pluralistic mode of thinking regarding health care system still exists in the minds of the people. In popular sector of medical science ayurvedic, homeopathic and a host of indigenous medical systems may find a reputed place. The experiences with biomedicine create in the people that they argue for searching the alternative. Alternative medicines have a great potentiality to become a medical system like biomedicine. Provided all the notions surrounding them are dispelled and more a scientific temperament is created in them.

References

Anderson, Robert, 1996. *Magic, Science, and Health: The Aims and Achievements of Medical Anthropology*, Fort Worth: Harcourt Brace College Publishers.

Barber, Hans A., Merrill Singer and Ida Susser (eds.), 2003. *Medical Anthropology and the World System*, London: Praeger.

Dunn, Frederick, 1976. Traditional Asian Medicine and Cosmopolitan Medicine as Adaptive Systems, *In* Charles Leslie (ed.) *Asian Medical Systems: A Comparative Study,* Berkeley: University of California Press, 133-158.

Chrisman, Noel J. and Arthur Kleinman, 1983. Popular Health Care, Social Networks, and Cultural Meanings: The Orientation of Medical Anthropology, *In* David Mechanic (ed.) *Handbook of Health, Health Care, and the Health Professions,* New York: Free Press, 569-590.

Leslie, Charles, 1974. The Modernization of Asian Medical Systems, *In* John Poggie Jr. and Robert N. Lynch (eds.) *Rethinking Modernization*, Westport.: Greenwood Press, 69-107.

Press, William L., 1980. Toward a Theory of Practice, *In* Elizabeth M. Eddy and William L. Partridge (eds.) *Applied Anthropology in America*, New York: Columbia University Press, 211-233.

Panikkar, K.N., 1992. Indigenous Medicine and Cultural Hegemony, *Studies in History* 8(2): 283-308.

Petersen, Alan and Robin Bunton (ed.), 1997. *Foucault, Health and Medicine*, London and New York: Routledge.

Nichter, Mark and Margaret Lock (ed.), 2002. *New Horizons in Medical Anthropology*, London and New York: Routledge.

Romanucci-Ross, Lola, 1977. The Hierarchy of Resort in Curative Practices: The Admiralty Islands, Melanesia, *In* David Landy (ed.) *Culture, Disease and Healing: Studies in Medical Anthropology*, New York: Macmillan, 481-487.

Sargent, Carolyn, F. and M. Johnson (ed.), 1996. *Medical Anthropology: Contemporary Theory and Method*, London: Praeger.

5

Health and Urban Poor

Sumita Chaudhuri

World Health Organisation (WHO) defines Health as a state of complete physical, mental and social well-being and not merely the absence of disease or infirmity. In a country like India, it is often said that proper health care facilities are not available everywhere and particularly not affordable by the poverty-stricken people. Under such a situation, the condition of the poor particularly the urban poor is quite critical as they do not get the pollution free environment like the rural poor has they often have to stay without a proper shelter, where basic civic amenities are characteristically lacking. Under such a situation, the plight of the urban poor is quite precautious. In this paper an attempt has been made to examine some of the health condition under the extreme impoverished limiting situation.

It may not be out of context to discuss briefly the background and situation of the urban\poor. The growing number of people living in slums and as pavement dwellers is intimately related to the process and pace of urbanisation in this country as a whole. Although the growth of India's urban population has not been very remarkable in recent years, the increase in terms of absolute numbers has been quite large. Certain trends are discernible which seem top link the rate and process of urbanisation to the pace of development in the rural sector, as well as to observed patterns of rural-urban migration of the poorer sections to cities within and outside the migrants' home state. There are really no accurate figures available regarding the exact number of people living in the slum or pavements in the major cities in India owing to the paucity of census data.

The total number of pavement dwellers or houseless population or beggars in four mega cities in India is only a fraction of the number of people living in slums. However they tend to be concentrated in certain areas of the city, and this, plus the fact that their every activity from cooking to bathing and sleeping is carried out in public view makes them far more visible than slum dwellers. Their problems are also obviously more severe as they have no privacy.

Regarding the social identity of this urban poor in all major cities in India, these are predominantly from lower castes and other disadvantaged communities. The percentage of lower castes among the urban poor is also significantly higher than for the population of the city as a whole. As Majumdar pointed out, "the urban poor are the same as those in rural areas—both lying at the bottom of the social structure and suffering from cumulative inequalities". Another very important point is that in the past, landless labourers usually migrated to other villages in search of work for earning when adverse condition prevailed in their home village (Gaugh 1960, Cohn 1955). This still happens, but the cities of India over the last decade provided important alternative sources of employment to these people.

Efforts made over the years for improving health standards have been partially neutralized by the rapid growth of the population. It is well recognized that population stabilization measures and general health initiatives, when effectively synchronized, synergistically maximize the socio-economic well-being of the people. Government has separately announced the 'National Population Policy 2000'. The principal common features covered under the National Population Policy 2000 and National Health Policy 2002, relate to the prevention and control of communicable diseases; giving priority to the containment of HIV/AIDS infection; the universal immunization of children against all major preventable diseases; addressing the unmet needs for basic and reproductive health services, and supplementation of infrastructure. The synchronized implementation of these two Policies—National Population Policy 2000 and National Health Policy 2002—will be the very cornerstone of any national structural plan to improve the health standards in the country.

In most urban areas, public health services are very meagre. To the extent that such services exist, there is no uniform organizational structure. The urban population in the country is presently as high as 30 per cent and is likely to go up to around 46 per cent by 2051. The bulk of the increase is likely to take place through migration, resulting in slums without any infrastructure support. Even the meagre public health services which are available do not percolate to such unplanned habitations, forcing people to avail of private health care through out-of-pocket expenditure.

This study on the beggars was done in an important religious place—Kalighat in Kolkata. The first study was conducted by me in early 1970, a restudy in 1987-88, 1999-2000 and again in 2008-2009. It was noticed from the different periods that there are some development like two schools for the beggar children, one run by Nirmala Niketan, and another by one NGO, but the basic amenities available for the poor was meagrely developed. The public sector health facilities in Calcutta seem largely used for emergency purposes. For all other care, private practitioners or pharmacists are used. A study by the Indian Council of Medical Research (1985) reported that 85 per cent of the people did not use the Maternal and Child Health (MCH) clinics in the area. They reported that lack of information and awareness of the services of the clinics was partially responsible for the low use. From this survey as well, it seemed that the residents had little encouragement or information as how best the community facilities can be utilized. These poor migrants live in small shanties or on footpath, in and around Kali Temple of Kalighat areas. Due to increase of land prices these shanties were demolished where these beggars used to keep mainly their belongings inside the shanties and not for staying or sleeping purposes. In this situation these people faced several problems like no privacy or security. This type of situation is very much acute for the female beggars as they face problem at the time of their monthly period or pregnancy. Most deliveries occurred in the hospitals. As statistic this can be seriously misleading. In hospitals serving the urban poor, the conditions in which deliveries occur are barely acceptable, in terms of cleanliness, equipment, and quality of post-natal care. Hospital deliveries, in themselves, do not necessarily reflect modern or even better conditions. Among the women, it was interesting to observe that the main reason for going to the hospital was that any post-natal services or supplementary feeding would be provided only to children whose births have taken place in hospitals or clinics. The literature was examined to see whether some light could be thrown on the quality of care and profiles of use.

The existing data on maternal mortality is unreliable for a variety of reasons and unfortunately, there are few maternal mortality studies on urban poor (Abouzhar and Royston 1991). Of the few that exist, two studies of Calcutta's hospitals deserve mention as those serving nearly exclusively the urban poor communities. Studies by Dawn (1972) and Chaudhuri (1976) estimated Maternal Mortality Rates (MMR) at 950 per 100,000 live births at the Nilratan Sarkar Hospital. They reported hemorrhage and hypertensive disorders of pregnancy as the two most important direct causes of this mortality, with anemia and hepatitis as the principal underlying causes. Similarly, Konar (1973) and Guha (1972) reported MMR as high as 850 per 100,000 deliveries at the Eden Hospital. The authors pointed out that most of the maternal deaths were in the lower socio-economic groups, occurring within 24 hours of admission and were linked to anemia caused by parasitic diseases. Both anemia and hepatitis are conditions that are particularly amenable to public health action and are relatively easy to control. Therefore, their presence as principal underlying causes of urban maternal mortality underline the weaknesses of the current public health care system.

When I visited this place to study the beggars in early 1970, female beggars gave birth on the footpath where they stayed and the elderly female beggars helped for the natal care. But now these people can get some medical facilities from the local government hospitals, but after discharging from the hospital they come and stay in the very unhygienic condition. Being neglected the urban poor have so far endured ill health to a great extent. Another point is that these people including the very young children face the tremendous pollution as their place of abode is very close to road side. The environmental condition is a significant determinant of the health risks to which a community is exposed. Unsafe drinking water, unhygienic sanitation and air pollution significantly contribute to the burden of disease, particularly in urban settings.

Regarding for the drinking water, there is no such arrangements; they collect from the roadside tap or from old well. From the very meagre available data, it was found that these people have chronic gastro intestinal disorder, disease of mouth teeth and gums as they do not wash properly or regularly. They have viral infection, stomach trouble especially during the monsoon, when some of the roads of this area are waterlogged. Due to poor sanitation system they get tremendous problem. In the early 1970, there were almost no toilet but nowadays there are toilets which are pay and use. These people usually do not avail these facilities as they have to pay even meagre amount, they are used to go on the bank of the river or some dirty areas. The female beggars usually use the old toilets of Kalighats dharmashala which are not at all regularly cleaned.

Pollution from a variety of sources was possibly one of the most important health risk factors in the slum areas. The potential for indoor air pollution and associated risks is indicated by the number of families who cooked and lived in same room. It is well known that the toxic constituents of kerosene and chemicals from the combustion of bio-mass fuel can cause acute respiratory infections (WHO 1991). Its health impact on children and old person who sleep and live in this area can be considered serious (Boyden 1991). As expected single roomed housing and use of bio-mass fuels were associated with poorer households particularly in the context of the slum dwellers.

Specific environmental risks and potential hazards associated with certain economic activities in the slums were exceedingly high. A few such examples may be cited here. In one slum, several small factories produced sulfuric acid, the vapours of which engulf the slum all day. In another slum, the main occupation is to recover and recycle metal from old car bodies which is then used to manufacture the telephone cables. At the final stage, the shifting process produces large quantities of fine metal dust which the workers continuously inhale. In another slum the principle occupation is the manufacture of wooden icecream spoons. The production process required the workers to dip the wood and bark by hand into heavily polluted water without any observable precautions or evidence of subsequent cleaning. Finally, street level habitation of the majority of the urban poor ensure the inhalation and continuous exposure to vehicle exhaust fumes known to be rich in carbon monoxide, oxides of nitrate and transient suspended particles, the human health effects of which have been widely studied and mentioned (Hamza 1989, WHO 1991).

The main findings of this chapter pertain to health aspect of urban poor and health specificities of the urban environment. The study is based on the fact the urban population form a substantial part of India and among them the poor are an increasing proportion. Their condition remains unrecognized as urban statistics are generally averaged over the entire urban population and thus misleading priorities in urban development. The survey confronted difficulties in estimates of the slum population and pavement dwellers that varied enormously. The principal findings were the following: the significance of the traditional sector in health care; the high cost of medical care and the high proportion of medical expenditures spent on medicine, the severe caloric and fat deficits among younger women and lactating mother; the tendency to spend less for medical care for women; and the penury of space and consequential exposure to pollutants (e.g. toxic fumes from biomass cooking fuels). In the analyses of these findings, several areas have been identified as practical priority issues that need to be addressed by policy-makers.

A major weakness in this type of survey has been the non-availability of correct data of health aspect for the pavement dwellers/beggars. The urban-poor are unequivocally a priority group and not only because they are the most disfranchised of all groups but also because they constitute a significant proportion of the global urban poor population. The pavement dwellers in Calcutta are a large and significant part of its urban environment and play a very important role in the city's developmental and growth potential, not to speak of the more fundamental considerations of social equity and justice. Special programmes through a comprehensive package of shelter, health care, and economic support programmes are urgently needed for this group. Mobile health care vans for evening or night services for these poor can provide care effectively to a large proportion of the poor, who would be otherwise unable to obtain them. In fact this was specifically suggested in National Health Policy 2002.

The neglect of the health conditions of pregnant mothers and of young women as precursors to conditions leading to maternal mortality also bears witness to the lack of serious efforts to improve health of women, even if it were just in the interests of the children they are to bear. The loss of a mother is possibly the greatest comprehensive disadvantage of any child. Programmes targeting the prevalence of risk factors producing life-threatening conditions at delivery should be addressed urgently, starting with better studies on the extent of and the underlying causes of maternal mortality. Maternal care could be improved by a system of upgraded traditional midwives (under some form of supervision), which would not only resolve the overload on understaffed, underequipped hospitals but also lower costs and provide cleaner and effective services.

The effective use of health care by women in the Calcutta slums as in India is closely related to her status and value in society. Urbanization has done little to change traditional attitudes and roles towards women among the urban poor. The alarming rates of nutritional deficits among young women, the high rates of wasted pregnancies, the preferential use of traditional medicine, and the lower levels of health expenditure for them, all bear testimony to the poor condition of the ordinary, low-income urban women. Much has been written about oppression and marginalization of women, less has been done to mitigate those circumstances. While there are admirable examples of action towards equal rights of women in the country, the rank and file, particularly in poorer states such as West Bengal, still live in oppressive conditions. The disease patterns of the urban poor reflect the problem of underdevelopment and industrialisation. The few studies that focus upon health problems of the urban poor demonstrate a prevalence of infectious diseases and malnutrition which is comparable to and often greater than that observed in rural populations. At the same time, however, the urban poor suffer the typical spectrum of chronic and social diseases. The magnitude of the health problems of the urban poor rarely emerges in city health statistics. This is either because the "unofficial" squatters and scanty town or slum inhabitants do not appear in the statistics or because their conditions are obscured by the enormous differences that exist between their status and that of urban elite. At the community level there is now evidence of relevant, constructive and hopeful approaches to helping the urban poor through primary health care. Although there are few analytical or evaluative examinations of such initiatives, it is possible to identify emerging trends such as the development of neighbourhood health programmes, the use of community health workers and attempts to link hospital services with community health action. It remains to be seen whether the health departments in any cities can bring about the coordination and support needed for the improvement of environmental and socio-economic conditions which are fundamental for improving health.

By the end of the century, half of the World's population will live in cities. Calcutta and other Indian cities will remain among the top of the list of the largest metropolises, despite the concentration of resources, the majority of the urban population in India will probably remain beyond the reach of critical services, unless urgent efforts are made. The situation of the urban poor today is appalling, not only in India but in many developing countries. To change their situation does not require new knowledge or technology but rather new approaches and the will to act in favour of the disfranchised for the well-being of all.

References

Abouzhar, C. and E. Royston, 1991. *Maternal Mortality: A Global Fact Book*, World Health Organization, Geneva.

Bhagat Ram, B., 2005. *Urban Growth by City and Town in India*, Paper presented in the Annual Meeting of Population Association of America at Philadelphia, USA.

Bose, Ashish and J. Bhatia, 1978. *India's Urbanisation 1901-2001*, New Delhi: Tata McGraw Hill.

Boyden, J., 1991. *Children of the Cities*, London: Zed Books.

Chaudhuri, Sumita, 2003. The Urban Poor: Struggle for Existence, *Journal of the Indian Anthropological Society* 38: 355-361.

CMDA Report: Electronic document. www.nzdl.org/cgi-bin/library/cig, accessed May 9, 2010.

Cohn, B.S., 1955. The Changing Status of a Depressed Caste, *In* Mckim Marriott (ed.) *Village India,* Chicago: University of Chicago Press.

Dawn, C.S. with N. Gupta and D.L. Poddar, 1972. Avoidable Factors in Maternal Deaths, *Journal of the Indian Medical Association,* 59(3):101-104.

Fauveau, V. with M.A. Koenig, J. Chakraborty and A.I. Chowdhury, 1988. Causes of Maternal Mortality in Rural Bangladesh, *Bull World Health Organ* 66(5):643-51.

Gough, K.E., 1960. Caste in a Tangor Village, *In* E.R. Leach (ed.) *Aspect of Caste in South India, Ceylon and North West Pakistan*, Cambridge: Cambridge University Press.

Hamza, Alavi and John Harriss (eds.), 1989. *Sociology of Developing Societies: South Asia*, New York: Monthly Review Press.

Planning Commission, Government of India, 2001. *Draft Approach Paper to the 10th Five Year Plan, 2002-2007*, Planning Commission, New Delhi.

United Nations, 2001. *World Urbanisation Prospect: The 1999 Revision*, Population Division, Department of Economic and Social Affairs, U.N., New York.

Victora *et al.*, 1988. The Operation of the Concept of Social Class in Epidemiological Studies, Sao Paulo: 22.

WHO, 1992. The Role of Health Centres in the Development of Urban Health Systems, *WHO Technical Report Series 827*, Geneva.

6

Socio-cultural Dimension of Health Care Practices: A Study among the Ao Nagas of Nagaland

Pranjal Boruah

Introduction

Health is man's natural condition, therefore, it is always a major concern of the community development and problems of health are the problems of national importance. The Government of India was a signatory to the *Alma Ata* Declaration, and the South East Asian Health Charter with the WHO for achieving the goal of "Health for All by 2000" (Sharma 2005). Though the rapid advances in the field of medical science in the last century have helped in reducing mortality, the morbidity has significantly increased. There are more people suffering from various diseases today than ever in the past. Pollution, poverty, lifestyle, food habit, social and personal stresses and many other factors have contributed to this sense. Health and social development cannot be separated from each other, and social sciences research is of much significance in health care planning.

Health of an individual as well as the community is largely influenced by social and cultural factors which are deeply interwoven with the social fabric of life. These factors have wide variation from one community to another and also within the community itself. The health problems need special attention in the context of tribal communities in India because of their settlements in difficult areas and circumstances. The health, nutrition and medico-genetic problems of diverse tribal groups inhabiting widely varying geo-climatic conditions present a formidable challenge for effective health care delivery. Similarly, the common beliefs, customs and practices connected with health and disease are intimately connected with the treatment of disease. Several studies reveal that socio-cultural and economic factors have tremendous impact on Health status of the tribal community (Bairathi 1991, Kar 1993, Pokarana 1994, Kar and Gogoi 1995, Kar and Barua 1997, Pandey *et al.*, 2001, Yadav and Sharma 2002, Medhi and Paul 2004, Ajala *et al.*, 2005, Biswas and Kapoor 2005).

Despite gradual expansion of modern education and increasing contact with the outside world, very often it is observed that the social, economic and cultural factors poise as barrier in availing of modern medicare facilities. Since the health care practices of a community are also prescribed its deep-rooted tradition like beliefs, customs, practices, literacy and prevailing health care facilities, therefore studies on socio-cultural correlated of the tribe will help to understand their health seeking behaviour which in turn will be helpful to plan interventions to improve their health status. Keeping all these facts and views in mind in the present study, it is proposed to attempt an appraisal of socio-cultural life and health care practices of the Ao Nagas, a major tribe of Nagaland in North-East India. Discussions have, by and large, been centred around the economic life, food habits, living conditions, health resources and utilization, maternal and child health etc., that prevail among the people.

The empirical data presented in this chapter has been generated through field investigation in three homogeneous Ao Naga villages, namely Lirmen, Yajang-A and Yajang-B in rural setting. All these three villages are located in an identical geographical setting i.e. under Japokong range in Mokokchung district, Nagaland but in differential accesses to modern health services. Standard anthropological tools were used in the collection of field data.

The People

The Aos, a major Naga tribe, are the principal inhabitants of Mokokchung district of Nagaland state in Indian Union. According to mythology of the Aos, they claim that their ancestors emerged from the stone (Jamir and Lanunnungsung 2005). The name Ao means went or went away (Aier 1990). They call themselves *Ni-so-meh* and

Sa-mai-na (Sen 1987). According to Ao traditional history they descended from Longterok (which means six stones). Nearby this place they first founded a village named Chungliyimti and settled there for a considerable period. In course of time they crossed the Dikhu river by cane bridge leaving others behind. The people, who went ahead leaving others behind, came to be known as 'Aor' or 'Ao', meaning going or gone. It is at Chungliyimti that they have their origin of history, culture and social set up.

Though the exact route of Ao migration is not known, from various cultural traits left behind it is believed that they came from Burma to Manipur, Manipur to present Chakesang area, from there to Yimchunger area and from there to Sangtum area where lies Chungliyimti they crossed to present place in the north-west of the state of Nagaland (Ghosh 1982). However, most of the scholars have agreed that the Nagas in general and so the Aos also have come from south-east of their present habitat. They have come from different places of Indo-China that is land between India and China, or from South East Asian Islands. They have got similarities of culture with Philippines, Indonesian, Melanesian and Polynesian people.

The Ao Naga belongs to Mongoloid stock. They speak Tibeto-Burman language and are divided into Chungli, Mongsen and Chungki section based on their dialect. They are endogamous and divided into several clans. They do not have any script of their own. Nuclear type of families is predominantly found among them. Inheritance is in the male line and in case of absence of sons, only the close agnatic male members inherit the property, particularly the landed property. Though originally animistic, under the influence of missionaries, the people have now embraced Christianity.

The Population

The total population of the village Lirmen is 624 (53.36% male and 46.63% female) which is distributed in 130 families and that of Yajang-A is 414 (53.14% male and 46.85% female) which is distributed in 101 families. The total population of Yajang-B is 130 (53.07% male and 46.92% female) which is distributed in 28 families. The average size of a family in Lirmen village is 4.8 and that of Yajang-A village is 4 and Yajang-B is 4.6. With regard to family type, it has been found that the Nuclear type (110; 84.61% in Lirmen, 83; 82.17% in Yajang-A and 24; 85.71% in Yajang-B) dominates over the Extended (2; 1.53% in

Lirmen, 2; 7.14% in Yajang-B and not a single one in Yajang-A) and Broken (18;13.84% in Lirmen, 18;17.82% in Yajang-A and 2;7.14% in Yajang-B) types. The literacy rate among the people of Lirmen village is 96.47 per cent (male 51.92%; female 44.55%) and that of Yajang-A is 89.13 per cent (male 48.06%; female 41.06%) and Yajang-B is 70.76 per cent (male 36.92% and female 33.84%). The main source of livelihood among the people is agriculture (59.29% in Lirmen village, 59.42% in Yajang-A village and 39.23% in Yajang-B village). However, there are few families who have taken up services (4.80% in Lirmen, 1.69% in Yajang-A and 1.53% in Yajang-B) and business (1.12% in Lirmen, 0.72% in Yajang-A and 0.76% in Yajang-B) either in lieu of or in addition to agriculture.

Economic Life

The people have predominantly agricultural economy. They are traditionally shifting cultivators. Although agriculture is the main occupation of majority of Aos, it does not confine them throughout the year. They are also engaged in other economic activities like raising vegetable gardens, cattle farming, poultry and livestock keeping, basket making, collection of wood both for the purpose of house construction and fuel, hunting and fishing. The daily expenses in a household are generally met from the cash earned through the sale of forest and jhum products. In a few households nearly all day-to-day expenditure is met with salary of the working members. Majority of the people do not have any savings and live at a bare subsistence level economy. Only a handful of the people enjoy a life better than those of the others because of the regular cash income earned in the form of salary. Thus the socio-economic condition of the people as a whole seems to have a negative influence on their overall health and well-being.

Food Habit

The staple food of the people is rice. The people generally take three major meals a day, i.e., early in the morning, in the mid of the day and in the evening without much restriction of the food items. They do not have any idea of the need of a balanced diet. People are fond of the flesh food (viz. meat and fish) and they believe that these foods contain all the required nutrients for the body. These items are not in regular menu and these are taken less frequently than vegetables. Ignorance of the need of additional nutrients during pregnancy, post-natal period and after prostrated illness etc., seem to be common feature among the people. Due to the nutritional deficiency, because of poverty, a number of diseases may originate among them. Anemia, general weakness and eye problem etc., are some of the frequently incident nutrition related diseases among the people. Except a few educated women, others are not concerned about the balanced diet of their children. The supplementary feeding is not different from the diet of the other family members and they also do not maintain any proper time schedule for feeding their babies.

Living Condition

The people by and large, are not very particular and conscious regarding the maintenance of a healthy surrounding as well as personal hygiene. They do not take bath regularly. Both men and womenfolk take bath only one time after returning from the jhum field. Frequent affliction by various types of skin diseases (e.g., scabies, boil, ring worm etc.) can also probably be explained in terms of their unhealthy living condition as well as lack of personal cleanliness. Proper toilet facilities are very important health factors as most of the diseases are borne from open field or *katcha* type of toilets. Among the people under investigations, it has been observed that except two households in Lirmen village who possess sanitary latrine, all the other households have *katcha* type of toilets. The people go to these latrines with bare foot and they do not use a separate cloth for it. They are also not conscious about the use of toilet soap after defecation. Though all the family possess housing facilities, it seems the standard of the house are far from being adequate. The houses are not provided with sufficient light and ventilation. As a result the smoke that billows from the hearth accumulated within different rooms and the inmates do not get the required free air and light. All these are believed to be detrimental for health and are likely to herald a number of diseases such as respiratory problem, lungs problem, asthma, eye problem etc. Since the people under study are widely distributed in the hills in rural settings, they totally depend on the river and spring water for drinking as well as for other purposes. This water is carried through the pipe or canal system towards the village area, where they usually have a big tank to store. All the people carry water in bamboo pipes from these tanks. Due to scarcity of water and as the tanks are far away from their individual houses, they also store water in iron drums and in the bamboo pipes for 3-4 days and these are not properly washed. The preserved water, however, mostly remains uncovered. Some households also possess overhead cemented tanks where they store the rain water. The only problem with the overhead tanks is that they do not clean the tank regularly so microbes get developed in these tanks. The households are not aware of this type of pollution and this resulted in some water borne diseases. Jaundice, Typhoid, Malaria are very common diseases among them.

Health Resources and Utilization

The prevailing health resources among the people under investigation may conveniently be discussed under two broad categories: modern resources and traditional resources. The traditional resources can again be divided into two types: magico-religious and herbal medicines. The people of Yajang-A and Yajang-B village by and large, take the services from both the resources depending on the nature and severity of the diseases. But the people of Lirmen village, mostly, take the service from modern resources. However, in some preliminary health problem, they take some indigenous herbal medicines.

In Lirmen village, there is a government dispensary with a pharmacist, one nurse and one midwife. The dispensary is a *katcha* type and where facilities of treatment for minor diseases are available. But infrastructure of the dispensary is very poor. The people of this village first consult with the pharmacist or nurse for their diseases and depending on the nature and severity of the disease they give medicines and if they are not cured even after using medicine, the people then go to Morioni, Dimapur, Mokokchung for better treatment. However, in initial stages of some diseases they try to cure by taking some indigenous herbal medicines. There is no any reputed traditional medicine man and magico-religious man in this village.

In Yajang-A village, there is one health sub-centre with one nurse and one midwife. The sub-centre is also *katcha* type and not in regular service. During the investigation it has been observed that in most of the time, the nurse is not available in the sub-centre and used to get transfer within a short duration. In this regard, the people of this village have to depend on modern health resources available in the nearest town for allopathic treatment. But there is a reputed herbal medicine man and a magico-religious man in Yajang-A village. People of this village mostly depend on these two experts, depending on their nature of the diseases. In case of harm of evil spirit and snake bite they approach the magico-religious man. For all other diseases, they first approach the herbal medicine man, as they believe that he can diagnose the actual disease and cure it. It has been reported that the medicine man could cure some diseases which are not cured by the modern medicines. Their economic condition is a factor, for which they approach the traditional medicine man. It is their assumption that if they go to modern practitioners they are to spend a large amount and sometimes even the patient is not cured. The traditional medicine man never demand any amount from them and most of the time, he gives free check-up. The medicine man diagnoses the case first and depending on the nature of the disease, he gives his prepared medicine. In case, the disease is not curable by him, he advises the particular case to take help from modern resources. Sometimes, in some minor cases, he prescribes the medicines to take from the pharmacy nearest to them. Thus, the medicine man serves both traditional herbal practices as well as modern allopathic practices.

In the village Yajang-B, there is no health sub-centre or dispensary. So, the people of this village go to the nearest town Haluwating and Amguri for Allopathic treatment. As their transportation facility is not good, they have to come on foot or have to hire taxi from Haluwating to reach these modern resources at the cost of Rs. 300-400. The people of Yajang-B village originally came from Yajang-A village and from same clan. Therefore, they by and large depend on the medicine man of Yajang-A. The people first approach to the herbal medicine man in time of their diseases. If the disease is not curable by him then according to his suggestion they take the help of other modern (allopathic) health resources where available. For snake biting, and wrath of malevolent spirit they take the help of magico-religious man of Yajang-A.

In order to have a quantitative idea, on the overall morbidity pattern and the type of treatment used among the people, primary data have been collected through house to house investigation in the villages under study. Depending on the knowledge and experience of the people, a list of 52 diseases along with the native terms could be collected (Table 6.1). The frequently incident diseases include fever, malaria, gastritis, dysentery, jaundice, liver problem, cold and cough, kidney problem, intestinal problem etc., and the relatively less frequent diseases include appendix, heart problem, injury, urinal problem etc.

Table 6.1: Distribution of the Diseases/Ailments Episodes Among the People under Investigation

Sl. No.	*Name of the disease/ailment (Local term, if available)*	*No. of afflicted person (%)*			
		Lirmen	*Yajang-A*	*Yajang-B*	*Total*
1.	Malaria (*Ramen*)	16(3.23)	36(7.28)	14(2.83)	66(13.36)
2.	Fever (*Yimra*)	6(1.21)	38(7.69)	1(0.20)	45(9.10)
3.	Gastritis (*Tartipen*)	40(8.09)	—	3(0.60)	43(8.70)
4.	Intestinal problem (*Tar tashi tak*)	25(5.06)	1(0.20)	—	26(5.26)
5.	Liver problem (*Temesen angoba*)	19(3.84)	6(1.21)	—	25(5.06)
6.	Dysentery (*Pokchi*)	6(1.21)	16(3.23)	1(0.20)	23(4.65)
7.	Typhoid (*Tuku tashi tak*)	10(2.02)	10(2.02)	—	20(4.04)
8.	Kidney and urinary tract problem (*Tezungjang*)	15(3.03)	4(0.80)	—	19(3.84)
9.	Cough (*Akutba*)	11(2.22)	8(1.61)	—	19(3.84)
10.	Stomach pain (*Pokcha*)	5(1.01)	10(2.02)	—	15(3.03)
11.	Sinusitis (*Teni tangpangba*)	13(2.63)	—	—	13(2.63)
12.	Respiratory problem (*Kurik*)	11(2.22)	—	1(0.20)	12(2.42)
13.	Jaundice (*Tasu*)	—	11(2.22)	1(0.20)	12(2.42)
14.	Mensturation problem	10(2.02)	—	—	10(2.02)
15.	Eye problem (*Tanuk angba*)	9(1.82)	1(0.20)	—	10(2.02)
16.	Anemia	9(1.82)	—	—	9(1.82)
17.	High blood pressure	9(1.82)	—	—	9(1.82)
18.	Gall bladder stone (*Backtsutem*)	5(1.01)	4(0.80)	—	9(1.82)
19.	Tonsilitis (*Tekong tezu tem*)	8(1.61)	—	—	8(1.61)
20.	Asthma (*Teku tepangba*)	6(1.21)	—	2(0.40)	8(1.61)
21.	Back pain (*Terem chain*)	6(1.21)	—	—	6(1.21)
22.	Rheumatism (*Teli chain*)	6(1.21)	—	—	6(1.21)
23.	White discharge (*Temesung aoba*)	6(1.21)	—	—	6(1.21)
24.	Dental problem (*Tuba angaba*)	5(1.01)	1(0.20)	—	6(1.21)
25.	Beri-beri	5(1.01)	—	—	5(1.01)
26.	Neurological problem (*Tezu tashidak*)	5(1.01)	—	—	5(1.01)
27.	Haemoglobin deficiency	5(1.01)	—	—	5(1.01)
28.	Tuberculosis	2(0.40)	3(0.60)	—	5(1.01)
29.	Headache (*Takolak angaba*)	3(0.60)	1(0.20)	—	4(0.80)
30.	Diabetics (*Chini tashitak*)	3(0.60)	1(0.20)	—	4(0.80)
31.	Lungs problem (*Tebokbok*)	3(0.60)	—	—	3(0.60)
32.	Bodyache	3(0.60)	—	—	3 (0.60)
33.	External injury	3(0.60)	—	—	3 (0.60)
34.	Appendisitis	2(0.40)	—	1(0.20)	3 (0.60)
35.	Scabis	3(0.60)	—	—	3 (0.60)
36.	Ear problem (*Tunarong angoba*)	1(0.20)	2(0.40)	—	3 (0.60)
37.	Diarrhoea (*Tupakeaa*)	—	3(0.60)	—	3(0.60)
38.	Leprosy (*Temangnang*)	2(0.40)	—	—	2(0.40)
39.	Mouth ulcer (*Tepang komu*)	2 (0.40)	—	—	2 (0.40)
40.	Boil (*Komu*)	1(0.20)	1(0.20)	—	2 (0.40)
41.	Worms (*Tapzen*)	—	—	2(0.40)	2 (0.40)

(Contd.)

(Contd.)

Sl. No.	Name of the disease/ailment (Local term, if available)	No. of afflicted person (%)			
		Lirmen	*Yajang-A*	*Yajang-B*	*Total*
42.	Neck gland enlarge	2(0.40)	—	—	2 (0.40)
43.	Ring worm	1(0.20)	—	—	1(0.20)
44.	General weakness	1(0.20)	—	—	1(0.20)
45.	Hair fall (*Ku tsukba*)	1(0.20)	—	—	1(0.20)
46.	Mumps	1(0.20)	—	—	1(0.20)
47.	Venereal disease	1(0.20)	—	—	1(0.20)
48.	Nasal bleeding	1(0.20)	—	—	1(0.20)
49.	Low blood pressure	1(0.20)	—	—	1(0.20)
50.	Vomiting (*Saktsuba*)	—	1(0.20)	—	1(0.20)
51.	Pneumonia Paralysis	—	—	1(0.20)	1(0.20)
52.	Panalysis	—	—	1(0.20)	1(0.20)
Grand Total (%)		308 (62.34)	158 (31.98)	28 (5.66)	494 (100)

Table 6.2 represents the village-wise distribution of the people according to acceptance of different medicare systems. It is seen from Table 6.2 that out of a total of 494 disease episodes, 370 (74.89%) people have resorted to modern medicare system whereas, 115 (23.27%) have taken up traditional one and 9 (1.82%) have gone for both the systems. Comparing the rates of acceptance of different medicare systems in the three villages, it has been observed that in Lirmen village utilisation of modern medicare system is more than the Yajang-A and Yajang-B village. But, in Yajang-A and Yajang-B village both traditional and modern medicare systems are used simultaneously.

Table 6.2: Village-wise Distribution of the People According to Acceptance of Different Medicare Systems

Sl. No.	Name of the Village	No. of Ailment Episodes (%)	Type of Medicare System		
			Modern (%)	*Traditional (%)*	*Both (%)*
1.	Lirmen	308 (62.34)	308 (62.34)	—	—
2.	Yajang-A	158 (31.98)	45 (9.10)	113 (22.87)	—
3.	Yajang-B	28 (5.66)	17 (3.44)	2 (0.40)	9 (1.82)
Grand Total (%)		**494 (100)**	**370 (74.89)**	**115 (23.27)**	**9 (1.82)**

Maternal and Child Health Care

Due to lack of proper health resources, the mother child health is also a problematic one. For knowing about pregnancy, women usually rely on their own diagnosis, in which the absences of periods, vomiting, feeling of hotness, nausea, weakness, greedy for sour are the key factors. From conception to delivery of the child the Aos by and large do not have any idea of medical check-up. They do not seem to be very much concerned about the necessity of some special care of the mothers' health. It is due to the non-availability of adequate health resources and health education among the people. The Ao women carry more of the work burden of the household and therefore have less time to seek out health care services making them disadvantaged relative to men in their access and utilization of health care services. However, a few educated women are found to take health check-up during pregnancy period from the physician of nearest town. Besides, the health centres are far away from their villages and it is difficult for them to cover a long distance, as the transportation facility is not sound. Most of them cover it by walk. In the villages under study, most of the deliveries are carried out at home by traditional midwives. Sometimes, a trained midwife or nurse is called if available. A woman is likely to be taken to a clinic or hospital when she has serious complications. Due to lack of proper health resources they cannot give proper health check-up to their children. As a result, the children die without getting timely proper health check-up.

An attempt was made to have a quantitative idea about the antenatal check-ups attended by the women and their place of delivery. In this regard, 60 married women respondents were considered from Lirmen village, 58 from Yajang-A village and 20 from Yajang-B village with an age grade 15-49. Table 6.3 shows the village-wise distribution of the women attending antenatal check-ups before delivery.

Table 6.3: Village-wise Distribution of the Women Attending Antenatal Check-ups

Sl. No.	*Name of the village*	*No. of women*	*Yes*		*No*	
			N	*%*	*N*	*%*
1.	Lirmen	60	7	11.66	53	88.33
2.	Yajang-A	58	4	6.89	54	93.10
3.	Yajang-B	20	—	—	20	100.00
Total		**138**	**11**	**7.97**	**127**	**92.02**

From Table 6.3, it is seen that in the villages under study out of 138 women, 7.97 per cent women went for antenatal check-ups before delivery, while 92.02 per cent women did not. Considering the villages independently it is seen from table 6.3 That in the village Lirmen, 11.66 per cent women went for antenatal check-ups before delivery, while about 88.33 per cent women did not. Similarly, in the village Yajang-A 6.89 per cent went for antenatal check-ups, while 93.10 per cent women did not. But in the village Yajang-B not a single women went for antenatal check-ups before delivery.

Table 6.4 shows the village-wise distribution of place of delivery. From Table 6.4 it is seen that out of 433 births, 93.76 per cent were delivered at home while 6.23 per cent were delivered at hospital. Considering the villages independently, it is seen from Table 6.4 that in Lirmen village, out of 189 births, 91 per cent were delivered at home while 8.99 per cent were delivered at hospital. In the village Yajang-A, out of 172 births, 96.51 per cent was delivered at home and 3.48 per cent were delivered at hospital. Similarly, in the village Yajang-B, out of 72 births, 94.44 per cent were delivered at home while 5.55% were delivered at hospital. Thus, it is seen that in all the three villages, the percentage of home delivery is maximum than that of hospital delivery.

Table 6.4: Village-wise Distribution of Place of Delivery

Sl. No.	*Name of the Village*	*No. of Women*	*Place of Delivery*		*Total*
			Home (%)	*Hospital (%)*	
1.	Lirmen	60	172 (91.00)	17 (8.99)	189 (100)
2.	Yajang-A	58	166 (96.51)	6 (3.48)	172 (100)
3.	Yajang-B	20	68 (94.44)	4 (5.55)	72 (100)
Total		**138**	**406 (93.76)**	**27 (6.23)**	**433 (100)**

Conclusion

The above discussion clearly brings out the differential in the health care practices among the Ao Nagas in Nagaland. The findings reveal that the Aos still have to subscribe their traditional medicare system as the modern medicare system is not accessible to them. Though the development of Christianity highly extended among the people and tries to improve their socio-religious-economic aspects but it is seen that the people are still behind in some aspects mainly in case of their health care practices. It has been observed that government health departments have introduced many needful schemes for the well-being of the society but these are yet to reach in rural areas. There is need of proper investigation and inspection to implement the government health schemes in these rural areas. However, to bring an overall development or improvement in health scenario of the people there must be provision of proper free and easy accessible of modern medical facilities. People should be educated and motivated for modern treatment so that they can come out from their traditional habits and practices and can maintain their proper personal hygiene and environmental sanitation. Health education programme for the women is highly needed to promote health awareness among them. This programme should give greater attention to the nutritional aspects as well as regular health check-up for pregnant women. Further, road communication is one of the major problems of the rural people; it should be improved with the help of new technology.

Acknowledgement: The article is a part of doctoral work which was supervised by Prof. Indira Barua of Deptt. of Anthropology, Dibrugarh University.

References

Aier, I.T.A., 1990. *The Religion of the Ao Nagas,* Jorhat: Assam Printing Works.

Ajala, O.A. *et al.*, 2005. Accessibility to Health Care Facilities: A Panacea for Sustainable Rural Development in Osun State South Western Nigeria, *J. Hum Ecol.* 18(2):121-128.

Bairathi, S., 1991. *Tribal, Culture, Economy and Health,* New Delhi: Rawat Publications.

Biswas, R.K. and A.K. Kapoor. 2005. Health Seeking Behaviour among Saharia A Primitive Tribe of Madhya Pradesh, *Indian Journal of Social Science Research* 46(3):249-260.

Ghosh, B.B., 1982. *History of Nagaland*, New Delhi: S. Chand and Co.

Jamir, N.T. and A. Lanunnungsang 2005. *Naga Society and Culture*, Jorhat: Borkatoki and Co.

Kar, R.K., 1993. Health Behaviour Among the Tribes of North-East India: A Profile. *Journal of Indian Anthropological Society,* 28(2):156-164.

Kar, R.K. and J. Gogoi., 1995. Health Culture and Tribal Life: A Case Study among the Noctes of Arunachal Pradesh, *In* R.C. Swarankar (ed.), *Indian Tribes, Health, Ecology and Social Structure,* Jaipur: Rupa Books Pvt. Ltd. 17-37.

Kar, R.K. and T. Barua, 1997. Morbidity and Health Behaviour: A Case Study among the Migrant Munda Tea Labourers, *Bulletin of Deptt. of Anthropology, Dibrugarh University, Dibrugarh*, XXV.

Medhi, B.K. and B. Paul, 2004. Health and Hygiene of the Nahs of Arunachal Pradesh, *Stud. Tribes Tribals* 2(1):23-27.

Pandey, G.D. *et al.*, 2001. Socio-cultural Aspects and Health Care in Pando Tribe of Madhya Pradesh, *J. Hum. Ecol.* 12(5): 391-394.

Pokarna, K.L., 1994. *Social Beliefs, Cultural Practices in Health and Disease,* New Delhi: Rawat Publications.

Sen, S., 1987. *Tribes of Nagaland,* New Delhi: Mittal Publications.

Yadav, A. and A.N. Sharma., 2002. Health Culture and Health Seeking Behaviour among the Semi-Nomadic Lohar-Gadiyas of Malthon Town of Sagar District, Madhya Pradesh, *J. Hum. Ecol.* 13(6): 431-435.

7

The Role of Food Habits and Social Practices in Understanding the Health Care of Kurichchan of Krishnagiri District of Tamil Nadu

Thambi Durai Thangavel and *Jesurathnam Devarapalli*

Introduction

The World Health Organization mentions *health as a state of complete physical, mental, and social well-being and not merely the absence of disease or infirmity.* In such a scenario health is not the mere biological; instead, it also means physical or biological, mental or psychological and social well-being. Once when someone speak of health; it was purely about the biological condition, and later psychological or mental state has also become a part of health. Only during the recent years the social health or the community health is taken into consideration as a part and parcel of health. There is an ample literature available on both biological and psychological health issues, but it is not so in case of community health, due to the reason that social factors are not considered as influencing biological well-being. In a mythical way, health is indeed a simple relay midway between the body and the mind (Barthes 1997: 24) and health is thus experienced through food only in the form of *conditioning*, which implies that the body is able to cope with a certain number of day-to-day situations (*ibid*).

Society is a collection of individuals, and thus now the collective health issues are in consideration in the name of social health or community health. Health is most important and integral part of life for any human individual, and thus from the beginning of human evolution the healthy can survive and those who can adapt to the environment can exist, underlining the Darwinian principle of *struggle for existence* and *survival of the fittest.*

So these two propositions will illustrate us the importance of health in the survival or existence of human individuals and of society as a whole. Every society invariably has its own health care system identified or created in the due course of time from the emergence of its culture or during the evolution of the same. But many of the so-called modern societies lost its health care system either due to the reason of the influence of modern medicine or lack of knowledge or interest in maintaining the traditional medical practices due to their felt inaccuracy.

Apart from this Anderson (1997: 80) mentions that in the Chou Dynasty, the Chou Li (rituals of Chou) prescribed that nutritionists be attached to the court as part of the highest class of medicinal personnel and this statement exemplify the importance given to food and they treat food on equal terms of medicine. To substantiate, Sen mentions that *you are what you eat* is the dominant theme of Indian medical and philosophical system (2005: 165). With this we can understand that the importance given to food items or food materials is equal to that of medicines. Further Anderson (1997) quote Arthur Kleinman and mentions about the Chinese traditional medical practice of altering food from that of the ordinary or usual one to some special category. He mentions that some foods are extremely strengthening; others are weakening, if eaten to excess (Anderson 1997: 81). Anna Meigs (1997: 95) cites Mary Douglas and state she consistently argued for greater attention to the social (as opposed to the nutritive and psychological) aspects of food and eating and Barthes mentions it as psychosociology of food: it is what might be called nutritional consciousness (1997: 25). And she adds through analysis of food and eating systems one can gain information about how a culture understands some of the basic categories of its worlds (1997: 100) here, the word *world* can be equated to culture or society, as how it understands the nature or the environment in which it persists. Meigs quote Mauss's work "The Gift" and mentions our feasts are the movement of the needle which sews together the parts of our reed roofs, making of them a single roof, one single world (Meigs 1997: 102). In her conclusion Meigs mentions that to eat a food, in the *Hua* conception, is not only an economic, social, and nutritive event but also an emotional and mystical one (Meigs 1997: 104). With this statement we can have an understanding that every society will not look upon things as same as others do. Apart from the commonness we have our own unique differences. As food eating is emotional and mystical for *Hua,* it plays a vital role in maintaining the structure or influencing in the formation or in the maintenance of culture. This influence and the emotional background are due to the environmental factors that have its influence in structuring the culture.

Ratzel was the first scholar to systematically study the relationships between the way of life of different groups and their habitats (Freilich 1967: 27). This is a thought provoking and an important viewpoint emerged in the discipline, due to the reason that the habitat/ environment has its own influence in the creation of any culture which is emerging amongst its purview. We are very much aware that many societies have its own taboo, and which are nothing but limited resources available in the habitat, when it is used extensively it may perish soon, so to maintain the presence and for its existence some such limited resources are considered and kept under the title *taboo* and people are strictly following it as a rule because that is a part of their culture that maintains the stability. For example, to a population which is subsisting on marine products will not have a fish or some other edible as their taboo or else the population will perish as they subsist on them. And again for *Toda* eating buffalo is a taboo as they are subsisting on them, so the influence of the environment/habitat in the formation of culture is much relevant. And Russel Smith argues that natural resources, climate, and accessibility are the stuff of which industry, trade, religion, national policy and to some extent civilization are made (1925: 3). In a simple sense these natural resources, climate and accessibility can be taken as habitat/environment and the industry, trade, religion, national policy are seen as culture and thus the statement exemplifies that how the habitat/environment influence in the creation of culture. To substantiate, Huntington states that the climate of many countries seems to be one of the great reasons why idleness, dishonesty, immorality, stupidity, and weakness will prevail (1915: 294). The climate is nothing but a part of the environment and that influences even the psychological factors according to Huntington apart from culture, or the culture leads to such a psychological factor as a result of such an environment.

Herskovits too mentions that the habitat of a people must be included among those influences that play on the formation and functioning of culture (1956: 156). So it is not the influence, it is influences and the habitat is one amongst many. For example the few other influences can be the neighbouring group, climate, resources, etc. but Herskovits emphasizes habitat as it has a predominant role. La Piere states that the belief in *sovereign influence of environment* has been widespread in space as well as in time. As a folk belief, it has frequently taken the form that people who live in the northern part of a given area are typically of stern and sturdy character, industrious and provident. Those who live in the southern section are characteristically easy going, indolent, talkative and of cheerful disposition (Cf. Freilich 1967: 26). It is more similar or adding strength to that of Huntington's view how the part of environment (here it is land section or arena) influence in the psychological character of a society. Freilich cites Mason and states that he designates twelve regions in North America as *Ethnic Environments* and summarized those non-human environmental factors like physical geography, climate, predominant plants, animals and minerals helps or influencing in determining cultural development (Cf Freilich 1967: 28).

In a similar pattern Meggars discusses differences in soil fertility, climate and other elements determine the productivity of agriculture, which, in turn, regulates population size and concentration and through this influences the socio-political and even the technological development of culture (1954: 802) takes place. Kroeber wrote that change in culture; due to natural changes in the environment undoubtedly occur. But this explanation for culture change has probably been propounded ten times for every actual case of such change (Cf. Freilich 1967: 30).

In the meantime certain opposive arguments are also staged by scholars, Herskovits is one among them, and he argued that if environment is indeed an important determinant of culture, similar environments should be inhabited by similar cultures. He also showed that similar cultures exist in different environments and that different cultures exist in similar environments (Cf. Freilich 1967: 29). Sanders added more strength to the supporters and stated that certain geographical conditions to be *crucial* to centres of civilization: the presence of a fertile soil; sufficient water for irrigation; easily controllable scanty plant cover; presence of a major river and a general deficiency of natural resources other than good agricultural land (1962: 36). The availability and accessibility of the resources in the given environment has to be taken into consideration and the utilization and the knowledge about the available resources and their pros and cons are gained in the due course will lead to the preference of the resources and leads to maximum utilization. This kind of resources preference and utilization can be termed as adaptation.

Each environment offers to human occupation a different set of challenges, and therefore a different set of alternate cultural responses may be expected.... In responding to such challenges, cultural response tends to take the path of greatest efficiency in the utilization of the environment (Sanders 1962: 34). This kind of cultural response or utilization is otherwise known as adaptation. For example, our houses are well ventilated with windows and doors, we just cannot imagine a house with a single opening, and it is highly impossible for us to live inside such a building. But think of *Toda* and their huts with just a small single opening and they are happily living inside that, which is nothing but a cultural response for a challenge of survival with a greatest efficiency, and such a cultural response is nothing but an adaptation. The environment monitoring practices of some indigenous and rural societies are significant in identifying ways to perceive the continuum of nature holistically, as opposed to trying to reduce complexity to a few measurable and controllable variables (Peloquin and Berks 2009: 533)

Biologists increasingly recognize that adaptive differences can arise through a variety of processes, including developmental adjustments and evolved learning abilities which may themselves be affected by experiential factors (Cf. Mulder 1987: 28). The experiential factors are nothing but, human-environmental interaction. This interaction forms the emic knowledge and leads to adaptation. The adaptive differences are due to the cultural impact or up to its set up of right and wrong. Unless people respond and adapt differently, everyone allover the world will be almost similar and there will be a heavy competition for survival. When the neighbouring communities have similar cultural features and subsist on the same resource, then among them a heavy competition will prevail and persist for their survival, and finally all the resource deplete at one fine morning and the obvious result is the expiry of the communities as their subsistence already went off. So to fit for the survival, the cultures adapt differently and respond differently, and struggle for its existence. Finally it results in occupying the unoccupied niche, and there a different culture emerges.

The adaptive significance can only be identified in environments that do not radically differ from those in which the species is presumed to have evolved (Cf. Mulder 1987: 25). Unfortunately not only few societies, but almost each and every society have changed its environment from where it evolved. So the adaptive significance cannot be found among the modern societies, so the wonderland/paradise for those who are thinking off to know about the adaptive significance will end up in pre-industrial societies, simply the tribals, who are isolated from the complex societies. But that fact is also a mere utopia, since culture is not static and out of contact with neighbouring cultures the possibility of having some change is always been there and this kind of possible changes are explained by diffusionists and out of acculturation too it happens. Mulder (1987: 28) states it as in studying the distribution of traits in contemporary human populations, we can examine only the potential on which natural selection could operate, were the traits faithfully transferring from parents to off-spring, but can make no claims as to whether traits are mediated by genetic or environmental factors.

In this position the question of this chapter arise, how food habits and social practices will help in understanding health. What is the relevance of the literature presented earlier with this chapter? To make it proper, first the answer is for the second question *the relevance of the literature*. The presented literature provide us with a better understanding and an image about what are the parts of culture and how it has been influenced by the environmental factors, and what all can be the possible factors should be taken into consideration. As well it exemplifies how scholars perceived and had views regard the fact, the influence of environment and its factors in the creation, maintenance and for survival for the culture.

Kurichchan

Before entering into the answer for the first question, let us have a brief introduction about the tribe *Kurichchan*. They are settled in Dharmapuri and Krishnagiri districts of Tamil Nadu. They are not the original settlers of that place; they are migrated from Mysore region. Their dialect is more similar to that of Kannada, the language of the neighbouring state Karnataka. They are a patriarchal and a patripotestal community, have moiety organization. They were hunters and gatherers, shifted towards pastoralism and currently engaged in settled agriculture and in minor phase engaged in the both hunting-gathering and pastoralism too. The study is conducted in the year 2007 in

Ispathapalli village of *Maradhanapalli* panchayat included in *Denkanikottai* taluk. *Krishnagiri* is a hilly area and it is above the mean sea level of from 300 m to 1400 m.

Food Habits

Though shifted to agriculture the practice of hunting, gathering and fishing have their sporadic occurrence. The staple food of the community is *Raagi* (*Eleusine coracana*), they prepare *Raggi Muddhae, raagi* ball and take it along with a dish made out of *Kollu* (*Macrotyloma uniflorum*). Every society has developed indigenous botanical knowledge through its dynamic interactions with its surrounding environment (Furusawa 2009: 147). As it is a hilly region, involving in intensive agriculture is difficult and both *kollu* and *raagi* are made available through dry cultivation. The influence of the environment, the climate as well land made them stick to the staple *raggi* and *kollu* for their survival. Here, the environment influences the people or the society to cope up with it and to design their culture accordingly. Earlier the *Gowda*'s (the headmen) consume rice, as they are rich enough to buy rice compared to that of the community members.

As mentioned they are occasional hunters and gatherers. They used *bill-ambu* (cross bow and arrow) to hunt, but in the current generation, many people are unaware about the working mechanism of bow and arrow. They prepare their own nets and *urulu* for rabbit and different type of nets for different fishes. They hunt wild boar, rabbits, hedgehog, and other small games which are available in the forest region. They catch birds with special prey captive they prepared.

They go for scanty seasonal fishing. They have prepared their own nets to fish and also, *kodamai* a basket like equipment to catch fish in streams and channels. Now-a-days they are initiated to settled agriculture, cultivate rice, vegetables, beans etc. scantily. The major cultivated crops are *raagi, kollu* and bean and all these three are dry cultivation crops as the landscape and climate permits only that, so accordingly these people adapted to the environment in which they are living as they could not bring in high technological interpretations. Trying for some other crops will show crop loss and low results and that will definitely create an impact, which sometimes may result in troublesome survival. So coping up with environment is nothing but adaptation and is so necessary for the problem less survival. Similarly, utilizing the available resources is also a kind of adaptation and making use of the available resources through the earnest possible way. Social practices are nothing but adaptations and this will lead to further usage according to the success rate and finally it will become our culture.

Their dietary pattern includes both vegetarian and non-vegetarian diet like that of most tribal population. Like most primates, humans are omnivores in the narrow sense of consuming both plants and animals (Harris and Ross 1987: 91), by definition; an omnivore is any animal that takes food from more than one tropic level (Milton 1987: 94). This omnivorous capacity is undoubtedly a phylogenetic characteristic—a part of *human nature* (Harris and Ross 1987: 91). Though they are omnivorous, their source of vegetarian and non-vegetarian diet is different. The vegetarian diets include *raagi*, *kollu*, maize, etc. and are cultivated from their fields. The non-vegetarian diet is obtained by hunting and fishing. And apart from the hunted animals they consume meat of cow and sheep they rear. *Gheeru* is the main sweet which takes place almost in all feasts (*Indu*). *Gheeru* is a sweet made out of water, jaggery, and with some pulses. In general they provide vegetarian feast at the community level. They consume everything cooked, both vegetarian and non-vegetarian; they don't have the practice of consuming raw. They use to cook inside their house, cooking outside is unusual for them. Firewoods are used for cooking, and mostly collected from the nearby forests. Their cooking vessels are made of mud; other utensils like spoon are made out of bamboo, and coconut shells. They prefer boiled food than that of fried ones, and fried food substances are unobvious and mainly tne cooking medium is water. Many elderly people have the practice of chewing tobacco, while cooking too; they won't mind in using it and is known as *gatti thool*. The important restriction or taboo they have is on hunted animals and not on the cultivated. Just before they go for a game hunt, they worship their deity *Mudhappa swamy* for a good game, and the lower jaw of the hunted game is offered to deity. They never consume lower jaw of any hunted game; the lower jaw is tied up in a rope and hanged in a tamarind tree near the sacred spot. The term *taboo* might usefully be reserved for aversions of a more sacred sort namely, those which are backed up by elaborated religious notions of obedience to the will of a deity (Harris 1987: 78). As a part of their pastoralism, they rear cows and sheeps, they consume the dairy products milk and curd and buttermilk too. The consumption of milk is very less whereas intake of curd or buttermilk is very obvious in the afternoon meal.

Social Practice

Social practices are helpful in maintaining the biological, psychological health, to state the social practices are nothing but cultural practices or issues performed, and practiced by a community or a society as a whole, that universe accept it as a right one and follows and maintains. These social practices are nothing but accepted rules and norms for the well-being of the society and to perform better and to fit for the survival. Since these things are practiced by masses, these are not found overnight, probably experimented, and has been accepted for the well-being. Consumption of food is also a social practice as we follow the societal norms in our day-to-day life and since it helps in maintaining our biological health. Medicine man is also contributing enormously in the maintenance of the individual's health as well society as a whole. To specify *Kurichchan* hunt *Udumbu* (*Varanus sp*) and collect its fat and melt it to oil and make use of it in treating the fracture.

Shamanism is also a kind of accepted social practice by the society to maintain the psychological health. Sorcery, witchdoctor, and shamans are the performers contributing a lot in the maintenance of psychological health of the society. In *Kurichchan* they have some belief systems and all those can be fit into at least to anyone of the abovesaid criteria. They perform *deepa saguna* and *sombu saguna* to identify the reasons for the mischiefs happening in an individual's life or in a family. *Sombu saguna* and *deepa saguna* or *vilakku saguna* are two different forms of sorcery performed by the magician or *manthirvaathi.* Either they are descendents of the earlier performers or their disciples. Except the tools they use *sombu* (a beaker) and *deepam* or *vilakku* (a lighted lamp) almost other performances are more similar. The performer face eastern side and then spread paddy grains in the floor and place either *sombu* or *deepam/ vilakku* accordingly for the *sombu saguna* or *deepa saguna.* The sorcerer starts moving the concern object *sombu* or *deepam* in all the directions and chant some spells. During this in a particular place the object become immovable and cannot be moved and again he chant spells and he is able to find the reason for the mischief. The performer will find the reason and inform the concerned person, and he suggests to provide some offerings to either deity or to some ghost or some suggestions will be given by him. The concerned person accepts and performs whatever is said by the sorcerer. In case of some diseases first the sorcerer asks the patient to go to hospitals for a week or so. At the time if it is not cured then they perform again and identify the proper reason like, curse of deity, or ghost attack, or some mischief aimed or so. To solve the problem the sorcerer asks to offer a fowl, or sheep, or a cow for that particular deity or ghost in an auspicious day. And after such offerings they believe that within a month all the problems will be solved. This is a way to maintain the psychological well-being. Obviously a type of adaptation out of mischief happening in his/her life, they may lose hope of survival, and at times of such a scenario, this kind of things appear as ray of hope. When the performer says that individual due to certain reasons the mischief happened and by making certain offering, you can get rid off the mischief and that offering would appease the deity or the ghost. Psychologically the individual feel better and he start to have hope and belief, soon everything will be fine. So apart from biological health, psychological well-being is also important and an adaptation for better survival.

The social practice of hygiene and the environmental support for that seems to be more important in the health aspects. So discussing about the hygiene and health practice is important and necessary. Hygiene starts from individual and ends up in community or society. When the individuals are hygiene, obviously the society too is hygienic. The simple and the best way to be hygiene are to take bath everyday. But it is not so in case of these people. They take bath in the nearby lake *seegadi*, twice or thrice in a week, and no special things are used to take bath, they bathe their cattle in the same lake and they consume the same water for the purpose of drinking, cooking, cleaning etc. There is no toilet facility in the settlement, so they do open defecation, after defecation, cleaning is also done in the same lake.

They don't have the practice of brushing, instead, they collect the urine of cow and goggle it. In the cooking practices also the maintenance of hygiene is very poor. The women folk, use beetle leaves as well tobacco even during cooking, and spit inside the home and beside over. The typical home of *kurichchan* is shown in Fig. 7.1. The premise of the *kurichchan* house consists of space for human and cattle they rear. As they are forest dwellers they have to take care of their cattle or else they will be attacked by wild animals and hence some portion of the house is allotted to cattle. As they are kept inside the house animals defecate inside the house. So the question of hygiene rises to the most. They don't do the cleaning very much, as a result lot of that mosquitoes, houseflies, and other insects are present almost everywhere inside the house and the settlement. Foul smell emanates from their dwellings. Clipping of nails is also not there, washing hands before food is also absent. They involve in all kinds of work and immediately turn for food. There is no special hygienic practice by them.

Societies accept values, norms, and follow them strictly, and that differentiates one society from other. A feature that is possible, right, and accepted by a culture may not be so for the immediate neighbouring culture and thus cultural relativism upholds every culture has its own reason for its activities and performances and thus looking at the activity or performance without cultural context it is not useful and cannot be understood. Every culture has its own context and reasons for its action, such an action performed by the actors are according to the need and necessity with the influence of the environment and finally that is what we mention as culture and that differentiates one from the other.

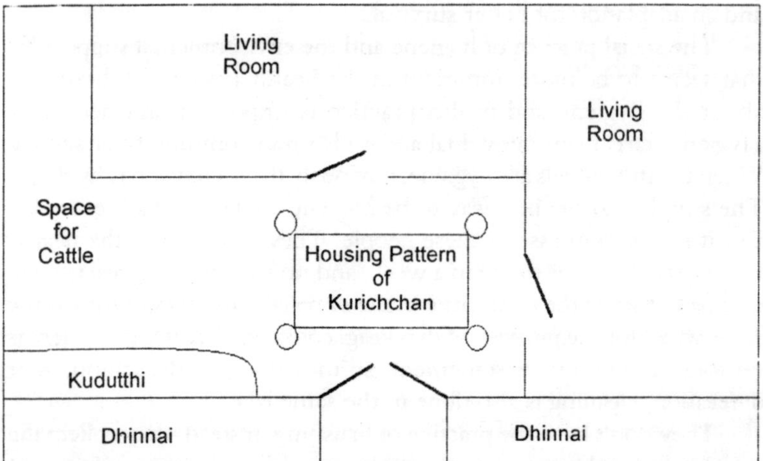

Fig/ 7.1: Typical House of *Kurichchan.*

Conclusion

With the context of Franz Boas, any activity has its own cultural context, either food, dressing pattern, marriage, and residence after marriage, family type, relationships, anything and everything. So with this, we can say the food practices what they have is not only to satisfy the biological need of appetite but beyond that to maintain the health and to make the survival possible. And making use of natural resources with the possible ways also be considered as an adaptive mechanism for better survival and well-being. Environment is one such important factor influencing culture and creates the context of survival. And only healthy practices are adapted and practiced and modified if necessity arises. Thus the food habits and social practices of *Kurichchan* help them to lead a life psychologically and culturally comfortable. But the biological health depends upon the kind of nourishment the food habits provide. The persons can be healthy only if they have all the nutrients—proteins, fats, carbohydrates, and vitamins in the required proportion. There is much relation between health and hygiene. When the body or some organ system is attacked by a pathogen (mostly due to the socio-cultural practices) it keeps on inflicting its harmful effects and ultimately destroying the health of the individual. Therefore, the slackness in any culture to accept and apply better technology to do away with environmental limitations may not be able to ensure the biological demands of the people.

References

Anderson, E.N. 1997. Traditional Medical Values of Food. *In* C. Counihan and P.V. Esterik (eds.) *Food and Culture: A Reader*, New York: Routledge, 80-91.

Barthes, R. 1997. Toward a Psychosociology of Contemporary Food Consumption. *In* C. Counihan and P.V. Esterik. (eds.) *Food and Culture: A Reader,* New York: Routledge.

Freilich, M. 1967. Ecology and Culture: Environmental Determinism and the Ecological Approach in Anthropology, *Anthropological Quarterly* 40: 26-43.

Furusawa, T. 2009. Changing Ethnobotanical Knowledge of the Roviana People, Soloman Islands: Quantitative Approaches to its Correlation with Modernization, *Human Ecology,* 37: 147-159.

Harris, M. 1987. Food Ways: Historical Overview and Theoretical Prolegomenon. *In* M. Harris and E.B. Ross (eds.) *Food and Evolution: Towards a Theory of Human Food Habits,* Philadelphia: Temple University Press, 57-90.

Harris, M. and E.B. Ross (eds.) 1987. *Food and Evolution: Towards a Theory of Human Food Habits,* Philadelphia: Temple University Press.

Meggars, B. 1954. Environmental Limitation on the Development of Culture. *American Anthropologist, 56*: 801-824.

Meigs, A. 1997. Food as a Cultural Construction. *In* C. Counihan and P.V. Esterik (eds.) *Food and Culture: A Reader,* New York: Routledge, 95-106.

Milton, K. 1987. Primate Diets and Gut Morphology: Implications for Hominid Evolution. *In* M. Harris and E.B. Ross (eds.) *Food and Evolution: Towards a Theory of Human Food Habits,* Philadelphia: Temple University Press.

Mulder, M.B. 1987. Adaptation and Evolutionary Approaches to Anthropology, *Man NS* 22: 25-41.

Peloquin, C. and F. Berks. 2009. Local Knowledge, Subsistence, Harvests, and Social-Ecological Complexity in James Bay, *Human Ecology* 37: 533-545.

Sanders, W.T. 1962. Cultural Ecology of Nuclear America, *American Anthropologist,* 64: 34-44.

Sen, C.T. 2005. *Food and Culture in India*, London: Greenwood Press.

Soler, J. 1997. The Semiotics of Food in the Bible, *In* C. Counihan and P.V. Esterik (eds.) Food *and Culture: A Reader,* New York: Routledge.

WHO. 2010. Official Website, Electronic document, http://www.who.int/hdp/en/index.html. accessed 20th February, 2010.

8

Suicide: An Anthropological Study at Sagar Block, West Bengal

Samar Kumar Biswas

The Sagar Block

Administratively, Sagar and Ghoramara group of islands belongs to the Sagar Community Development Block[1] in the district of South 24-Parganas, West Bengal (Bandyopadhyay *et al.*, 2004: 238). The Sagar Block lies between 21°37′-57′N, 88°02′-11′E. The geographical area of the islands was 219.26 km^2 (Bandyopadhyay, 1997b: 51). The deltaic Sagar and Ghoramara Islands of the Kakdweep sub-division falling within the administrative control of the district of South 24-Parganas situated at the mouth of the Hooghly River. This block, or the two islands were completely separated at a distance of four km. from each other and the main land too was treated as merely remote regions in this country. It is to be mentioned that before 1904, these two islands were attached and then it was known as Sagar Island.

It was bounded by the Hooghly on the West and by the Baratala or Channel Creek on the East, and on the South by the Bay of Bengal. The Northern extremity of the island, which was about 25 miles long, was called Mud Point (Ghoramara) and was the site of a telegraph station. Here the Sundarbans steamers leave the Hooghly and passed down Channel Creek on their Eastward route through the Sundarbans. At the south-western angle of the island stands the Sagar Lighthouse, which was built in 1808, and the Southern sea face was the site of the

Great Bathing Festival of Ganga Sagar (O'Malley 1914, reprinted 1998: 325-326).

This area held an important position from the environmental and ecological point of view. Tidal flooding, river fluxes, waves, long-shore currents, sea-level changes, cyclones[2] and storms as well as the environmental hazards are dominant physical processes that continually modify the course in a short and long-term basis (Das, 2006: 31-32). The natural environmental hazards (NEH) may be a natural event which is harmful to human and cannot be considered by them to be part of the normal state or condition of the environment; its potential for harm varies with the physical parameters of the event as well as the socio-economic conditions and political situations of the place of its impact (Bandopadhyay, 1997a: 21). There are a number of factors such as salinity[3], sandy soil, soil erosion[4], the daily intertidal flow or tidal waves, natural hazards i.e. floods, storms, cyclones etc. threaten the ecosystem as well as human life at Sagar and Ghoramara Islands.

Cyclone, Storm, Flood, etc.

Cyclones in West Bengal which were of oceanic in origin heat the coasts of Medinipur and South 24-Parganas four to five times a year (Mandal, 2004: 117). To such cyclones the area, Sundarbans was peculiarly exposed on account of its position at the head of the Bay of Bengal, and its records showed that, though they occurred at irregular intervals, these violent storms were far more destructive of lives and properties than either droughts or floods (O'Malley 1914, reprinted 1998: 168). Such storms not only damage crops, destroy hutments but also take a heavy toll of domestic cattle and human life (Chakrabarty, 1995: 31).

The great atmospheric disturbance affected the whole delta and in this regard it was more serious particularly in case of Sagar and Ghoramara Islands. The natural environmental hazards like cyclones, storms, tidal waves and floods seriously affect the daily life of the people of Sagar Block in different ways such as breaking of coastal embankments, destruction of crops, erosion of farmlands and settlements and damaging of other properties conspicuously. Storms and floods occurred in 1823, 1833, 1838, 1856, 1864, 1867, 1868, 1869 and 1871 on such scale as to seriously affect the crops and lives (O'Malley, 1914; Pargiter, 1934; and Mandal, 2004). In June 1823, a storm destroyed the roads, embankments and tops on this Island. Only ten years latter again in May 1833, the great gale and inundation occurred which destroyed the almost all progress of Sagar Island (Pargiter 1934, reprinted 2002: 338-341). The Sagar Island was submerged to a depth of ten feet, and the whole population of 3000-4000 souls is said to have perished (O'Malley 1914, reprinted 1998: 178). Storm occurred in June 1842, October 1848, and again in June 1852, which inflicted serious damage at Sagar Island (Pargiter 1934, reprinted 2002: 339). The serious cyclone took place on 5th October, 1864, which swept over the Sagar Island with full force and wrought great havoc (Pargiter 1934, reprinted 2002: 341). As might be expected, by far the greatest loss of life occurred on Sagar Island. The storm-wave entered at Sagar Island where it was eleven feet above the level of the land. At Sagar Island the wave destroyed nearly every building, and left scarcely any living creature on the Island. The few people that did escape saved themselves either by climbing trees, or by floating on the roofs of their houses, which the wave carried inland. At first it was reported that 90 per cent of the population had perished, but it was afterwards ascertained that 1488 persons survived on Sagar Island, out of a population before the cyclone of 5625 souls (Hunter 1875, I [I] reprinted 1998: 266-267). Again on 1st and 2nd November, 1867 occurred another cyclone and high tide which caused great damage to the lives, crops and reduced the area under cultivation from 31,190 to 2750 *bighas*[5] (Pargiter 1934, reprinted 2002: 338-341). The cyclones of 1869 also affected the crop production very much (Mandal, 2004: 14). The most serious floods occurred in 1900, 1904 and 1907. There was tremendous rainfall, which caused floods and damaged nearly the whole of the standing crops (O'Malley 1914, reprinted 1998: 171-72). The cyclone which appeared in the district occurred on 17th October, 1909; it caused considerable damage to houses, trees, crops and cattle (O'Malley 1914, reprinted 1998: 178).

The cyclonic storms and floods in 1942, 1971, 1973, 1976, 1981, 1988, 1996, 1997 and 1998 destroyed the crops, lives including man and cattle, houses and other properties in a great degree. The 1976 cyclone that crossed Sagar and Ghoramara Islands on 11th September was the latest major event till now. Its maximum surface wind speed reached 130 to 148 km h^{-1} (Pant *et al.,* 1978 in Das, 2006: 16). This storm caused a widespread damage in the coastal area of West Bengal and adjoining state Orissa (Das, 2006: 16-18). The cyclonic storm that took place in November 1988 was caused by depression that blew over the area causing large scale devastation all around (Chakrabarty, 1995: 31). Three of the most destructive tropical storms that ever affected Sagar Island occurred on 21st May, 1833 (near about 7000 people died),

5th October, 1864 (4,137 i.e. 73.6 per cent people died) and 17th October, 1942 (Bandopadhyay, 1997a: 25).

Soil Erosion

In 1851-1855, the total area of the island was 284.55 km^2 which was reduced to 219.26 km^2 in 1997 (Bandyopadhyay, 1997b: 52-53). In fact, in the last 142 years (1855-1997) due to soil erosion 65.29 km^2 (23%) area of land was washed away and became a part of the river/sea. In this way the Ghoramara mouza was detached from main Sagar Island in 1904-05. Originally, the Sagar Block covered nine Gram Panchayats (GPs) with 46 mouzas, but due to soil erosion three mouzas viz. Khasimara, Lohachara and Bisalakshmipur were eroded and during study there were only 43 mauzas. Mostly in waterfront mouzas due to soil erosion and breaking of embankments the influx of saline water and loss of cultivable lands adversely affected the agricultural production. Even among the 27 coastal mauzas of Sagar Block, 23 were constantly being reduced due to soil erosion among which nine mouzas lost more than 25 per cent of their original extension (Bandyopadhyay, 1997a: 27-29; 1997b: 52-53; Bandyopadhyay *et al.*, 2004: 253-254; and Maity, 2005a: 25). Due to this fact it was noticed that, 1462 families were displaced only from Ghoramara Island which is itself a mouza, and among them only 447 families got rehabilitation. It is obvious that the people had to fight continuously against the adverse environment and it has and will have serious effect on the local people and on their economy and life. In this context, the committed suicide was also reported. In this study these are the important area of enquiry.

Research Methodology

Considering the effect of natural hazards and particularly the soil erosion on human life, the present study was conducted in four villages at Sagar Block, Sagar Island and Ghoramara Island. To investigate and study in details, two categories of villages viz. (A) settled villages and (B) rehabilitated villages were selected. In this regard two settled villages, namely Bagpara and Khasimara were situated in the most affected area and were located at completely isolated tiny (1 km. radius) island, Ghoramara which is itself also a mouza[6]. Basically Ghoramara Island was an isolated island nearly at a distance of four km. away from the Sagar Island and mainland too and considered as a Gram Panchayat

(GP)[7] consisted of six villages under Sagar Block, district of South 24-Parganas in West Bengal. The other two rehabilitated villages, Jibantala and Kamalpur were located at Sagar Island[8] where the people of erstwhile Ghoramara Island got rehabilitation very recently, 1992-1999. Further in regard to village selection on the basis of soil erosion three types of villages were considered such as (i) less eroded, (ii) highly eroded, and (iii) fully eroded. In this context the village Bagpara was comparatively less affected than Khasimara village in respect of soil erosion and property damages; whereas the rehabilitated people who lost their land and property completely due to soil erosion and later got rehabilitation in other two villages of Sagar Island, were the early inhabitants of different villages of Ghoramara Island.

Principally, primary and secondary sources of information, evidences as well as data related with attempt to suicide or suicide were collected in two different ways from Sagar Island and Ghoramara Island of Sagar Block. In this regard except the suicide record of hanged cases, all other concerned data of all the villages of the Sagar Island were collected only from the indoor admission register of Sagar Rural Hospital during the period of 10 years 8 months (2.1.1997 to 27.3.1998; and 17.7. 98 to 28.12.07 = 10 years 8 months and 8 days). In case of Ghoramara Island, particularly data related to attempt to suicide or suicide were collected only through ethnographic field survey followed by the methods of case study, interview, focus group discussions (FGDs). The selected interviews were taken from the committed persons if survived or the concerned family members or in case of non-availability from other close kin members or neighbours who were well aware about the facts.

Effect on the Studied People

Mouza, Village and Land: Natural calamities and soil erosion mostly affected Ghoramara mouza where 55.01 per cent (1992) area of land was already eroded and became a part of the river. In this regard Bagpara[9] village was less eroded whereas Khasimara[10] village was highly eroded where 96.89 per cent area of land was washed away and now a part of the river; and except a very few, the land of the people of rehabilitated villages were fully eroded when they lived at Ghoramara Island. Due to continuous environmental degradation around 89 per cent studied families lost their main resource, the land, and it was in average 16.02 *bighas* per family and in total 5412 *bighas* at Ghoramara Island. It is noteworthy to mention that the agricultural land ownership pattern was seriously affected and the land ownership got limited to only 193 (50.66%) families whereas in the past it was 342 (89.76%) families.

Shelter: Considering the consequences of environmental degradation the house erosion was well observed. Around 87 per cent of the families faced the house erosion; and the families of rehabilitated villages were the worst victims of house erosion earlier at Ghoramara Island. Further, around 40 per cent families faced this disaster for thrice and more. It was reported that the number of house erosions faced by the people of rehabilitated villages were much more than the people of settled villages implying more insecurity and distress. It was noticed that only at Ghoramara Island, nearly 15 per cent of the studied families had not any own homestead land. Again, the homestead land holding pattern of around 73 per cent of the families was quite poor and it was not more than 0.5 *bighas*. Further in settled villages around 85 per cent families had the only one roomed house each. Meanwhile 136 (35.70%) families got rehabilitated at main Sagar Island but those houses were constructed very poorly and each family was given single room accommodation where the space was not enough.

Agriculture: Agriculture was the worst affected component of environmental degradation. The land erosion, cyclone, storm and excessive rain cause damage to crops. Loss of agricultural pursuits due to environmental degradation was noticed among the studied people. All the 199 (100%) agriculture practiced families were affected in various ways at Ghoramara Island. All the agriculturist families at Ghoramara Island lost their crop production due to flood caused by breaking of embankment and natural calamities. Among them, crop production was reduced due to only soil erosion in case of 97.41 per cent families. The soil erosion reduced the dependency on agriculture. Further due to soil erosion, 195 (98%) families lost a large amount of agricultural land, in some cases the total land was eroded and as a result both the amount of agricultural land and the agricultural productions were largely reduced.

Fishing: On account of shrinkage of working scope in agricultural sector the people tried to survive from the surrounding marine resources including *hilsa* fishing and later on *meen* (tiger prawn seeds) collection. As an alternative economy, highest percentage of families (35.70%) was primarily involved in fishing. But in this regard they were facing a lot of problems because it was noticed that the boats of twenty fishing families were destroyed by storm and tidal wave. *Hilsa* and other marine fishing were already diminished. *Meen* collection was also on the wane. Further in the rehabilitated villages the opportunity of fishing was very rare and thus around 62 per cent families had to go to Ghoramara Island for pursuing their fishing by covering a distance of 26 kilometres day in and day out. The entire alternative economy, fishing was going to decrease for which they had to face a lot of problems to maintain their livelihood. As a result of soil erosion, they were displaced and due to displacement the scope of earning through fishing got reduced to a great extent. Ultimately, they earned a little from this source and somehow could maintain their livelihood as there was no other better alternative.

Day Labour Work: Due to non-availability of working opportunity in agriculture and fishing sectors many of them were engaged in daily wage labour works and it was noticed that primarily around 21 per cent family depended on it. Continuous soil erosion resulted in gradual degradation of cultivable land and thus the produced crop from their agricultural land and related earning were reduced. The labourers who were dependent on agricultural works could hardly manage their works and for a considerable period of time, they had no work and earning. With the erosion of land, the scope of agriculture and related works were reduced and thus the people were suffering from several problems to maintain their minimum livelihood. The environmental degradation reduced the chances of getting good wage earning scope in the studied area. Thus if land degradation occurs in a place the possibility of getting wage related work attached to farming is reduced. So, environmental degradation has direct negative correlation with the wage earning activities.

Further, environmental degradation causes land loss due to excessive rain and salinity of sea water makes land uncultivable. As land was lost due to soil erosion and in the rehabilitated villages, the villagers hardly had any cultivable land. Moreover owing to this recurring crop failure a famine like situation was happened. Thus the agro-based economy was severely hit by soil erosion.

Income and Indebtedness: In spite of their hard struggle, per head average monthly income was not more than Rs. 357.38. Meanwhile, the daily income of an individual of two settled villages was Rs. 14.01 and in rehabilitated villages it was only Rs. 7.83. As a consequence of poor income they had no other alternatives than to face utter hardship to manage common minimum livelihood. Due to repeated environmental degradation, the people lost their agricultural land and their houses several times. Consequently owing to the break up of river embankment and influx of saline water their cultivated crops got damaged and their agricultural land lost its fertility. As a consequence, their agricultural productions and several related works suffered a major set-back. Ultimately it forced the concerned people to get enmeshed in the web of loan in various ways. It was reported that they had to face difficulties to maintain their livelihood with such poor income and nearly 63 per cent families were compelled to be indebted. The amount of loan was varied from Rs. 700 to Rs. 25,000.

Food: The repeated natural hazards and continuous soil erosion had seriously told upon the scope of the people to accumulate their food. Considering the food taken by the people, it was noticed that in the rehabilitated villages, around 80 per cent families could manage food with utter hardship and they consumed it with delicacy of pulses and vegetables rarely. The protein like fish, egg and meat were almost absent in their food. Further, nearly 48 per cent families could consume food for once or rarely twice a day with only rice, salt, chilli and infrequently pulses and vegetables. Animal protein was simply mere dream to them. It was noticed that due to lack of natural resources and economic scarcity, most of the studied people had to face utter constraints to meet their hungriness even sometimes they had to remain on an empty stomach for the whole day. Hence the soil erosion, other natural calamities and environmental changes adversely affected the backbone of the food and nutritional chain of the concerned people in both the situations.

Further in most of the cases, due to lack of earning scope they failed to provide the minimum requirements to the family members. This situation turned into regular quarrels and conflicts among themselves and neighbours too. This overall situation generated an adverse impact on the family members and in the concerned society.

Defeat, Depression and Suicide: Despite their hard work and struggle in their daily life they could hardly accumulate common minimum livelihood. The continuous environmental degradation made them unstable regarding their inhabitation and shrank their scope of primary occupation as well as income. Ultimately, it hampered their social and psychological development and personality formation. They were trying a lot to cultivate crops but the repeated natural hazards had resulted in all of their efforts to turn into vain. On the other hand, when they went to deep-sea fishing called as *sabar*, in some cases they could not return alive due to thunder-storm, cyclone etc. and its consequent resultant factors. Thus the common people were always in a psychological fear that at any moment they may loss their economic resources or even their life but they had no way to redress it.

Soil erosion, flood, salinity and cyclone had far reaching consequences in the context of the studied population. When land was lost the economy was disturbed, when houses were eroded the shelter was affected and all these contributed to uncertainty and unstability in their socio-economic life. The nature and change and adverse consequences depended on the degree and nature of soil erosion which had a varied influence on the villagers. The uncertainty created tension and conflict leading to self-destruction or killing. The continuous fear and pressure of insecurity and uncertainty affected their mind seriously. The responsibilities, duties, social burdens and the state of indebtedness made them psychologically ill and in most of the cases it turned into mental depression which ultimately agonized them. In this regard, an individual could not find any sort of alternative to cope up with this situation or to redress their problem. Sometimes to get rid of the situation they often accepted the psychological defeat without having any sign to improve the situation in their life rather more deterioration possibly engulfed them and death was considered as the best possible alternative to redress these worldly problems. In this context poison taken by the people in different ages mostly for suicide was a common phenomenon in the studied area.

In this regard it was known from the office records of Sagar Rural Hospital that in between the time span of nearly 10 years 8 months (1997 to 2007), 1368 people of above 4 years consumed poison to commit suicide only at Sagar Island. Among them the percentage of female was higher (61.99%) than the male (38.01%). In this context it is to be mentioned that at Sagar Island the highest percentage of people (76.83%) attempted to suicide in between the age group of 10-34 years. Further, it was noticed that the trend was more in case of female. It was observed that the attempt to suicide or suicide particularly among the females was highest, 255 (30.07%) in between the age group of 15-19 years. In case of male, the attempt to suicide or suicide was highest, 264 (50.77%) in between the age group of 15-29 years. Besides the hospital records, a huge number of committed suicides were taken place on account of hanging at Sagar Island but it was not possible to collect as those were the matter under police station.

Again, the data related with attempt to suicide or suicide or similar type of death at Ghoramara Island were not recorded in the office register of Sagar Rural Hospital because the concerned people of Ghoramara Island went to the Kakdweep Sub-Divisional Hospital of mainland, more convenient to communicate. To know the situation as well as root cause of suicide or attempt to suicide, a detailed study was conducted on the entire Ghoramara Island/mouza, covering six villages with a population of 5236 (Census, 2001). The concerned study reveals that during the period of 1991 to March 2008, total 41 persons, among which 22 (53.66%) males and 19 (46.34%) females took an attempt to suicide or similar type of death by several means. Among them 9 (21.95%) and 2 (4.88%) cases took place at the studied Bagpara and Khasimara villages respectively; whereas the rest 30 (73.17%) incidences took place in other four villages of the Ghoramara Island.

Case Study-1

A class V standard 22 years old house wife, Sita Kayal, by caste Namasudra lived at Roypara village, Ghoramara Island who committed suicide in July, 1991 by hanging.

Family Background: Sita Kayal was the wife of Bikash Kayal and they were the inhabitant of village Roypara, Ghoramara Island. Their house got eroded three times along with the entire three *bighas* of their agricultural land. In their family there were six members, including Bikash and his wife Sita, a daughter, two unmarried brothers and his widow mother. Earlier they were dependent on agriculture but due to land erosion they had to depend on fishing, day labouring or like that. His father died in 1990 and after one year, in 1991, his wife, Sita hanged herself. Basically Sita's mother-in-law, namely Bharati Kayal was the stakeholder of the earned wealth and without her permission nobody had any right to spend a little bit even in familial discourse and Sita had to depend totally on her directions. In such a situation, often Sita was thrashed with abusive words and quarrel by her mother-in-law and brother-in-laws. Basically it was connected with the issues related with food, money and shelter as well as other daily needs. Ultimately, it became almost a daily routine in her life. Even her husband, Bikash was not in a position to protect his wife or restrain his mother from such offensive words.

Incidence: In such condition once in a day of July in 1991, due to the occurrence of severe flood, Sita and Bikash went to fetch the drinking water at a long distance. Further Sita cooked the items for lunch but unfortunately those were not up to the mark and it turned into an outburst with severe quarrel between Sita and other family members. After that they took lunch except Sita. During afternoon around 3:30 p.m. when there was no member in the house, Sita closed the door from inside and hanged herself with rope and expired. Actually, Bikash was the only earning member of the family and quarrel as well as familial conflict was a matter of their daily routine. Particularly Sita was always insulted and deprived to get her common minimum requirements and they regularly treated her with abusive languages and utter negligence.

In case of female it was mostly due to their insecurity in several aspects. It is to be mentioned here that except very few all of them were married and quite at that early age they had to do several works along with household chores. These females coming to new family as wife had to adjust and adapt with new members and new socio-cultural situation. But they could not always withstand these due to extreme crisis and poverty and it created chaos and conflict and often it crossed the limit of their tolerance level and ultimately to get rid of the unfamiliar circumstances sometimes they tried to commit suicide as the ultimate alternative.

Case Study-2

Gurupada Maity, son of Badal Maity was a twenty year old married man having III class standard education. He resided at Mandirtala village, Ghoramara Island. By caste he was Mahiswya and earned from agriculture, day labour works and fishing. He committed suicide and expired in 1995 by consuming poison.

Family Background: During the period of incidence, the concerned family comprised of nine members such as Gurupada and his wife, one child and his parents, three unmarried brothers and one unmarried sister resided at Mandirtala village, Ghoramara Island. Marriage of his two sisters was arranged in 1988 and 1991. Their four *bighas* of agricultural land was eroded and later they had four *bighas* of agricultural land and for maintaining their livelihood along with agriculture they had to depend on fishing, day labour works and van-pulling outside the village. Gurupada was a van-puller and he was the prime earner of the family. He was always under tremendous economic pressure. Father, Badal Maity always nagged to Gurupada regarding money. In 1993, Gurupada got married and in 1994 he had a child. Further, in 1994, his father, Badal Maity helped his eldest son-in-law with an amount for financial support which was mainly taken from Gurupada forcibly. Afterward, in 1995 the family had to face a major set back due to damage of crop by flood. Thus, the continuous increase of familial demand and fulfilment of the livelihood requirements for all the family members were rapidly being risen up. Under these circumstances Gurupada was repeatedly pressurized by the family members, and his tolerance level was unable to bear up the pressure.

Incidence: The quarrel had become a daily familial routine and one day Gurupada was severely thrashed by the other family members. He took poison and expired.

In the context of male, there laid a continuous pressure of earning mostly imposed by their family. The guardians as well as the prime earner of the families had to face a lot of problems to maintain the livelihood of their families. Because the scope and resources of earning became quite abandoned and it was mainly due to soil erosion, salinity, natural hazards and so on. As a result, they failed to provide common minimum requirements to their family members like wife, children, parents and other members. Eventually, the continuous conflicts and chaos hampered their mental peace repeatedly. The entire situation created severe dissatisfaction because of their inability to execute material requirements of their family members which made them frustrated and sometimes to get relief from the pressures and inability to fulfil the demand of family members and other inconveniences they chose suicide as the utmost destiny.

Furthermore, at Sagar Island, the people who had taken the poison, among them, nearly 11 per cent people expired. They used different poisonous substances whatever they got at hand. Their depression and anger was so furious that around 84 per cent people used strong toxic compounds to get rid of this depression or like that; whereas rest of the people used several poisonous seeds and poisonous liquid compounds like acid, petrol, kerosene etc. for this purpose. Meanwhile at Ghoramara Island, amongst 41 (100%) cases of attempted suicide, 6 (14.63%) cases were under investigation; around 56 per cent people had taken poison and the rest were died by hanging. It may be added here that out of total incidences, only 16 (39.02%) people could escape the death, while around 61 per cent people expired.

Moreover, it was known from the study of 41 cases of attempt to suicide or suicide or similar type of death at Ghoramara Island that in

40 (97.56%) cases the families lost their landed properties due to soil erosion and hardly had any resources. These sorts of incidences were mainly due to shrinkage of earning scope caused by repeated environmental degradation including soil erosion, high salinity due to low pressure of fresh water, storm and cyclone which resulted in emergence of continuous uncertainty in the life of the people. The poverty, frustration and conflict in the families were increased and when it became unbearable, people attempted suicide. Furthermore, it is to be noted that the root cause of those attempts to suicide or suicide were several quarrels, conflicts and tension mainly the resultant factor of insecurity, uncertain economy as well as extreme poverty and frustration caused by environmental degradation. Thus, suicide or conflict was not only an individual or familial or community matter, rather it was the consequences because of environmental degradation.

References

Bandyopadhyay, S. 1997a. Natural Environmental Hazards and their Management: A Case Study of Sagar Island, India, *Singapore Journal of Tropical Geography* 18(1):21-45.

——1997b. Coastal Erosion and its Management in Sagar Island, South 24-Paeganas, West Bengal, *Indian Journal of Earth Science* 24(3-4): 51-69.

Bandyopadhyay, S. with D. Mukharjee, S. Bag, D.K. Pal, R.K. Das and K. Rudra. 2004. 20th Century Evolution of Banks and Islands of the Hugli Estuary, West Bengal, India: Evidences from Maps Images and GPS Survey, In S. Singh, H.S. Sharma and S.K. De (eds.), *Geomorphology and Environment,* Kolkata: ACB Publications, 235-263.

Chakrabarti, S.P. 1995. *Twilight and Dark Life in a Sundarban Village*, Calcutta: Das Gupta and Co. Pvt. Ltd.

Das, G.K. 2006. *Sunderbans Environment and Ecosystem,* Kolkata: Sarat Book Distributors.

Hunter, W.W. 1875. Reprinted 1998. *A Statistical Account of Bengal,* Volume I, Part I, 24-Parganas, Calcutta: Govermment. of West Bengal.

Maity, J. 2005a. *Sagardwip* (in Bengali), Kolkata: Standard Printing.

Mandal, A. 2004. *The Sundarbans: An Ecological History,* Kolkata: Readers Service.

O'Malley, L.S.S. 1914. Reprinted 1998. *Bengal District Gazetteers,* Calcutta: Government of West Bengal.

Pargiter, F.E. 1934. Reprinted 2002. *A Revenue History of the Sundarbans,* Volume-I, (From 1975 to 1870), Kolkata: Government of West Bengal.

Notes

1. **Sagar Community Development Block** or 'Sagar Block' or only 'Sagar' which is consisted of two distinct populated islands namely Sagar Island and Ghoramara. Presently Sagar Block is consisted of 43 mouzas under nine Gram Panchayats in South 24-Parganas of West Bengal.
2. **Cyclone**: An atmospheric system characterized by the rapid inward circulation of air masses about a low-pressure centre, usually accompanied by stormy, often destructive weather. Cyclones circulate counter clockwise in the Northern Hemisphere and clockwise in the Southern Hemisphere.
3. **Salinity**: A measure of the quantity of dissolved solids in ocean water is salinity. The total salinity of sea water sample can be determined by measuring only the chloride ion concentration following the relationship-Salinity (ppt) = 1.80655 × Chlorinity (ppt). The unit expressed of salinity is parts per thousand or ppt.
4. **Erosion**: The group of natural processes, including weathering, dissolution, abrasion, corrosion, and transportation by which material is worn away from the Earth's surface.
5. ***Bigha***: A local unit for measuring land. It varies from one-third of an acre to almost one acre. The standardized *bigha* in West Bengal is 14,400 square feet, which equals 1,333.33 square meters or roughly one-third of an acre.
6. **Mouza**: A mouza is the geographical expression of a unit of landmass for revenue settlement and revenue collection, whereas, the village is a human settlement within a mouza with strong social bond. Within a mouza there can be thus more than one village. And, at the same time there can be even one village belonging to two contiguous mouzas.
7. **Gram Panchayat (GP):** Gram Panchayat is the primary unit of three-tier Panchayati Raj Institutions in the state of West Bengal. Under three-tier system of democratic decentralization, Gram Panchayat is the apex body at village level as the third-tier which is the Panchayat organization for a collection of villages.
8. **Sagar Island** is also four km. away from the main land. The only Sagar Island is consisted of 42 mouzas under 8 Gram Panchayats in Sagar Block of South 24-Parganas in West Bengal.
9. **Bagpara** was one of the villages consisting of six villages under Ghoramara Island/Mouza/Gram Panchayat. At that time 55.01 per cent area of the total mouzas was washed out. But separate area of land erosion of any of the six villages of the mouzas was not mentioned. But it was observed that some portion of the Bagpara village was eroded.
10. **In earlier Khasimara** itself was a mouza of 9.65 km^2 (1922-1923) area of land and village too under Ghoramara Gram Panchayat. But due to continuous erosion 96.89 per cent (1992) area of its original extension

was washed away in the sea and the existing part was too endangered considering the facts of its vulnerability. Even then the Government authority officially did not mention the existence of the mouza anywhere and declared the mouza was completely eroded. But 77 families were still living in the Khasimara Village.

9

Death in Homeland is Sweeter than Life in Elsewhere to the People of Jadugoda

Soma Bandyopadhyay

Introduction

Man is able to adopt himself with specific environment and to shape their living according to the convenience of environmental condition. Even then if environment itself is being modified for so-called human welfare, it becomes tougher enough for man to bear it with.

"**Science**"—whether it is a boon or a curse, is a debatable question. Scientists always argue that scientific discoveries are always made for human welfare but some of the scientific discoveries sometimes bring even human survival to a cross road. Man demands scientific upliftment for their benefit, but that should not be in exchange of human life. Scientific discoveries and its application should consider several factors related to human existence. Among these factors environment probably gets the highest priority. Application of science should not only be eco-friendly but it should be human existence—friendly in true sense.

Scientific discoveries having negative impact on human existence are good in number but probably nuclear research is in the summit. Radioactive elements used for nuclear research have prolonged effect on Nature.

Jadugoda, east Singbhum, Jharkhand, India, about 40 kms. from Jamshedpur is a rich source of uranium ore. Since British regime mining of uranium was a common practice in this area. The Uranium Corporation of India Limited (UCIL) was established in 1967 as a public sector enterprise, under the administrative control of Department of Atomic Energy (DAE). UCIL started its operations in 1968 at Jadugoda with uranium ore mining and a processing plant each of 1,000 metric tonnes per day (MTPD) capacity. The processing plant at Jadugoda has been expanded and presently the overall processing capacity of the uranium mill is 2090 MTPD after opening of new mines at Bhatin and Narwapahar.

UCIL claims that their activities are thoroughly environment friendly. Two types of wastes—liquid and filtered solids depleted in uranium—are generated in ore processing. This neutralized slurry is classified and coarse fractions are pumped back to the mines as back-fill. The fine particles are pumped to the tailing ponds, where the slime settles. The clear liquor is decanted off and sent for treatment. In Jadugoda the first tailings pond was constructed in the nearby valley around 1 km away from the tailings treatment plant. After this pond got filled up, two more ponds were constructed. UCIL authority admits that ore mining and processing would have some impact on the environment. The authority is making effort to ensure that the effect on environment is minimum and it remains below the specifications provided by the national and international expert bodies.

UCIL declares that 'The Environmental Survey Laboratory' collects the environmental samples and

- monitor the water samples of streams and rivers passing through Jadugoda.
- analyze the samples of groundwater, soil, grass, vegetables, aquatic organisms.
- measure Gamma radiation and environmental radon in and around Jadugoda.
- evaluate the natural background environmental gamma radiation up to two kilometres.

UCIL may perform this environmental monitoring periodically but common people inhabiting the surrounding areas have no way to gather any information regarding outcome of this periodical monitoring. UCIL never arrange any awareness camp or anything else alike, not even bother to publish the report to let people know how safe their environment is after mining and processing of Uranium ore. The common people who are suffering deadly, undoubtedly has the right to have proper information according to the Right to Information Act.

Observation

Since 1990 reports are coming out in different journals, periodicals and newspapers of national and international fame that people residing in different villages near Jadugoda mine are suffering from some physical abnormalities. Considering the nature, frequency and hike of abnormalities the researchers are now convinced that these are the impact of radiation. Initially this consideration was restricted among the researchers but gradually several social workers and NGOs have gone through the reports. They have generated awareness among the ignorant tribal people. Presently people are convinced that they have invited their sufferings by giving their homeland to the ***Diku*** (outsiders).

UCIL representatives are of different opinion. UCIL claims that the technological devices used for processing of uranium are of international standard. In Narwapahar mine the underground output per man shift is about 1.9 tonnes, which is considered to be the best in the country. Dr. Ashok Mohan (Technical Adviser, DAE) and K.K. Beri (Director, Tech, UCIL) conveyed the message that—

> "UCIL is well aware of its responsibilities to ensure that there should be least impact of its activities on environment. The regular monitoring indicates that the impact on environment because of UCIL's operation is negligible. With its safe and environment friendly operations, UCIL could be a role model for other industrial units to follow."

Two different views create a confusing situation. Who are right! People like Sumitra Soren (30) of Tilaitand near Jadugoda who has lost her three kids soon after their birth, Ramdeo Kalindi (45), a temporary miner suffering from a mysterious ailment and has lost his son Tapan Kalindi (22) suffering from the similar ailment, Sudarshan from Dungridih who does not respond to any external stimuli and a lot facing different abnormalities, or the learned experts like Dr. Ashok Mohan, K.K. Beri, Dr. R. Gupta (C & M.D., UCIL) and many others!

On August 30, 1999, the Indian Supreme Court issued notice to the Union Government on a PIL seeking direction to take steps to insulate people living in the vicinity of Jadugoda uranium mine (*Indian Express*, August 31, 1999).

Dr. Sanghamitra Gadekar, a scientist measuring the radiation level with a Geiger counter found that the boundary wall of a school, constructed by UCIL has a radiation level ten times higher than the acceptable level. Dr. Sanghamitra Gadekar, says, "International standards allow a yearly exposure of 100 millirem for persons working in the nuclear industry." However, the readings taken by Dr. Surendra Gadekar, a nuclear physicist, near a vent from the underground mines was as high as 5,851.68 millirem a year, which is 58 times more than permitted limit. (*Times of India*, October 2, 2001).

On September 4, 2000, the Indian Supreme Court admitted a petition seeking direction to the UCIL to take stringent measures at the Jadugoda uranium mines (*The Hindu*, Sep. 5, 2000)

Nalin Verma, Patna based special correspondent of *The Statesman* reports in 2004 that more than 16 per cent of the children born in the villages within 5 km. radius of Jadugoda mine die within a year of birth. Ghanshyam Birulee, President, JOAR (Jharkhandis Organization Against Radiation) reported Nalin Verma that 47 per cent women of 15 villages around mining area undergo automatic abortions and 6 per cent of the children born in these 15 villages are handicapped. Mr. Birulee also claimed that it is hard to get anyone living beyond 60 years in any of these 15 villages. Nalin Verma also reports that the Environmental Committee of Bihar House visited the area and made three major recommendations like—

- Evacuation of people living with 5 km. radius and their proper rehabilitation.
- Use of covered pipes and drains for carrying nuclear wastes.
- Use of notice board highlighting radioactivity hazards.
- Formation of expert medical team.

Verma reports that UCIL simply ignored all the recommendations.

On April 15, 2004, the Supreme Court of India dismissed the PIL on the hazardous impact of the uranium waste disposal by the UCIL, at Jadugoda. The Supreme Court hold that in view of affidavit filed by the Chairman, Atomic Energy Commission, that adequate steps have been taken to check and control radiation arising out of uranium waste, the Court do not see any merit in the petition and accordingly it has been dismissed (Harsh Kapoor, *SAAN*, 12th May, 2004).

On 15th July, 2004 an open interactive discussion on uranium mining and its effects was arranged by KSU, MPHRC and HESPO. In this discussion Mr. Praful Bidwai, eminent columnist stated that the radiation uranium gives out are invisible, intangible but does enormous damage to the chromosomes, and added that the notion—'low dose of radiation is safe' is very wrong. Opposing the UCIL representative's view that very low dose of uranium is sent to the tailing ponds, Mr. Bidwai reported that the tailing ponds retain 85 per cent of the original radioactivity. In the same discussion Dr. R. Gupta, C & M.D., UCIL talked about the beneficial role of uranium and stated that anything done for development of a country has some risk so the fact of uranium radiation should not be exaggerated.

The UCIL has been awarded ISO-14001 certification from M/s. TUV of Germany. Eminent doctors from Tata Memorial Hospital, radiation experts from Bhaba Atomic Research Centre have surveyed the nearby area of Jadugoda mine and found that the congenital limb abnormalities were due to genetic disorders and gross malnutrition (*Times of India*, December 22, 2004).

Contamination Exists

Contamination surely exists around Jadugoda uranium mine. If uranium is exploited and is left on the surface of the earth, pollution will be generated. Moreover, if unmanageable tailings are positively used for the construction materials of the building or the road, contamination will be expanded further. However, according to Koide's investigation, contamination centering on tailing ponds seems to have not spread yet broadly. Since two villages, Dungridih-1 and Dungridih-2, are in contact with the tailing pond, soil is polluted and the air-gamma dose is also high. On the other hand, in the villages including Tilaitand those are not directly in contact with tailing ponds the air-gamma dose is not high. In addition, the soils of these villages were not contaminated by tailings. The result of this investigation is summarized below.

1. The contamination from the uranium mine has spread in Jadugoda.
2. The amount of air-gamma dose exceeds 1 m Sv/y in the villages, and reaches 10 m Sv/y around the tailing ponds.

3. The circumference of tailing ponds is polluted with uranium. The strength of the pollution in the tailing ponds is 10 to 100 times higher than the place without contamination.
4. No. 1 tailing pond has contamination of cesium. This fact shows that radioactivity was brought from another polluted source that was not uranium mine.
5. Especially Dungridih that is in contact with the tailing pond has high contamination. However, other villages have not contaminated seriously yet.
6. Radon emanated from tailing ponds etc. spreads contamination.
7. Mine-tailings used for construction material spreads pollution.
8. Product uranium is dealt with carelessly and has fallen in environment.

Nutritional status of different villages exhibits the fact that nutritional abnormality prevails irrespective of distance of a village from Jadugoda. 300 patients suffering from eight serious diseases have been examined. The diseases are—Tuberculosis, Congenital abnormality, Physical deformity, Infertility, Cancer, Skin problems, Phileria and abdominal diseases. In most of the cases especially in case of Tuberculosis, Cancer and Infertility those patients were selected who has consulted with a registered physician and they have diagnosed the disease. This frequency has direct relation with the distance of the village from Jadugoda mine as well as the tailing ponds. Patients' occupation is also important in the regard as frequency varies in relation to occupation.

The diseases, taken as parameters are the most frequent among the patients of different villages. But this analysis clearly depicts that the diseases which may be caused for radiation is more frequent among the patients of nearby villages. Maximum number of Tuberculosis patients is found in Bango, Dungridih and Chatijkocha. All the three villages are situated aside tailing ponds where according to Koide's analysis air is contaminated with high gamma dose. Tuberculosis has direct relationship with gamma dose (Shannon and Amelia 2002). Another important factor to be mentioned is 38 per cent of the total patients suffering from tuberculosis are working or retired employees of Jadugoda mine or mill.

Maximum frequency of congenital abnormality is found in Ichara, Chatijkocha and Dungridih. All the three villages are located nearer to

Jadugoda mine and the tailing ponds. In Ichara 59 per cent patient having congenital abnormality is within the age range of 0-7 years. Congenital abnormality has a very little to do with malnutrition. 87 per cent of the children having congenital abnormalities are normally nourished. This may be due to some abnormality in their genetic configuration. Since 1945 eminent scientists have proved on different occasions that radiation has a direct effect on gene. So this possibility cannot be thoroughly overruled as these children has born and going to be brought up within an environment where radioactive contamination possibly exists.

Patients having some physical deformities are of highest frequency in Dungridih followed by Ichara and Bango. Mostly children within 12 years are suffering from these abnormalities which may indicate cumulative effect of radiation. Maximum number of couple having no children are found in Ichara and Bango. In 73 per cent cases husbands are working in Jadugoda Mine or Mill. Those who have gone through medical check-up, husbands are found to be faulty in this regard. Miners believe that for a person, working in Jadugoda mine or mill for two years it becomes difficult to have a child.

Conclusion

Whatever be the cause, people of Jadugoda are suffering from different diseases. They are not getting proper treatment. They have a very little knowledge about the consequences of radioactive contamination. People who are working in Jadugoda are earning money in exchange of their own as well as their family members' lives. They are working with minimum facilities and UCIL projects itself as a growing organization which plays an important role in our national development.

The miners of Jadugoda do not get the facilities which they deserve as a part of their human right. People who were there at the time of initiation of Jadugoda mine can recall those facilities which UCIL has promised to provide. They are cursing themselves for inviting the ***Diku*** (outsiders) in their ***Disham*** (homeland) who has ditched them.

- They are not provided with proper duty uniform.
- They are exposed to a radioactive environment at a stretch for eight hours which should be maximum thirty hours in a week.
- Miners deserve one litre milk per day supply of which is presently stopped by the UCIL authority.
- For protecting dust deposition the miners should intake

sufficient amount of molasses but the Jadugoda miners are not fortunate enough to have it.

- Though the people are serving a leading organization of the Government of India but UCIL does not take any responsibility of the workers after their retirement. They don't have any provision of pension or medical aid after leaving their job.
- UCIL promised to provide rehabilitation or financial compensation to those tribal landowners who were forced to handover their fertile cultivable land for the construction of tailing ponds. But these poor landowners are presently living in the middle of nowhere.

People of Jadugoda are realizing that their sufferings are going to cross the limit. They are losing their air to inhale, land to cultivate and water to sustain. But still they are not ready to leave their ***Disham*** (homeland). They have started protesting against the activities of UCIL, they are placing their demands regarding their right to live to the UCIL authority. They are doing their best unitedly not only to lead a safe life but also to regain their ***Disham*** (homeland) free of troubles. If one considers their demands this emotion towards ***Disham*** will come forward. The **Kol** inhabitants of Jadugoda area cognize the movement as a venture to get their crop varieties back. They are seen to be very emotional while thinking about those paddy varieties like ***Chandrakanti baba*** which was of high yield and good taste. The **Oraon** inhabitants are missing those singing birds in the jungle which could not survive in the polluted air of Jadugoda. They want to live with all those they have lost, but they have to stay in Jadugoda as they cannot leave their place of birth, the place where they have grown up and the place which has got immense emotional attachment with their ecological niche. They have now decided to protest against the UCIL activities at their level best and their culture fashioned their cognition in such a way that the people accepted the fact that **Death in Homeland is Sweeter than Life in Elsewhere.**

References

Edward Gordon 1992. Uranium the Deadliest Metal. *Perception Magazine*, 10(2): 334-343.

Indian Express 1999: Aug. 31, p. 5.

Kapoor, Harsh. 2004: *Jadugoda case and Supreme Court Judgment.* SAAN, India. 12th May.

Koide, Hiroaki. 2002. The Investigation on Radioactive Contamination around Jadugoda Uranium Mine. http//www.j.rri.kyoto-u-ac.jp

The Hindu. 2000: Sep. 5, p. 2.

Times of India. 2001: October 2, p. 9.

Times of India. 2004: Dec. 22 Page 11.

Shannon, V.R. and Amelia N.G. 2002: Emergent Pulmonary Infections, In Jim Yeung and C.P. Escalante (eds.) *Oncologic Emergencies,* Canada: BC Decker Inc. Ontario, 249-256.

10

Child Worker and its Effect on Health: A Study on Stone Crushing Sector

Biswanath Gan

Introduction

Health is wealth so runs the proverb. The word health has its origin from the word *hal* meaning safe and sound. Hence, dictionary meaning of health is "the state of being hale and sound in body, mind or soul especially from physical disease or pain". Thus the health of man or of a nation is a concept which requires recognition that well-being depends upon attention to all the key social, political and economic variables that affect the life of man. A more recent and increasingly used definition is contained in the constitution of World Health Organization "health is a state of complete physical, mental and social well-being and not merely the absence of disease or infirmity".

The socio-cultural complexity of human life affects to a large extent, health habits and practices of a community. The rigidity of these acts as a barrier in the adoption of innovation. Nutrition, sanitation, hygiene, immunization, etc. which form important aspects of health are either not accepted or totally rejected because of social pressure in a community. These formulate the strength of indigenous medicine and are deterrents to the acceptance of modern medicine. Therefore, it becomes imperative to know health related socio-cultural practices to formulate policy for health promotion, health protection, early diagnosis and treatment of disease, limitation of disability and rehabilitation (Rizvi 1991: 13-14).

Concerning health, the child health is regarded as a serious highlighting issue because a large number of children in our society are deprived of getting their necessary health facilities and mostly suffer from numerous health hazards due to child abuse and especially the working involvement of children into hazardous sectors is perhaps a major obstacle to enjoy the highest attainable standard of health.

Child worker is a problem of the whole world and it is more acute in the poor countries belonging to the Third World, mainly due to economic backwardness of the families. Thus, economic reason moves the whole family to work as a production unit. The children also get engaged in such work by any means. In the rural areas the children belonging to the poor agro-based families generally work with their family members. On the contrary, in the sub-urban/urban slum areas, most of the children of the poor families do work either with their family members or individually, or under any person on daily wage basis or on monthly basis (Biswas 2006: 27). The prevalence of child labour has been more or less in all periods of time, though varied in its nature and dimension, depending on the existing socio-economic structure of society (Punecha 2006: 1). Today children form a sizeable section of the labour force in several areas of employment. Though child labour is a global phenomenon, its incidence is more acute in the less developed countries. It has been rightly observed by the ILO that child labour is essentially a problem of development. It is a phenomenon deep-rooted in economic and social conditions. The exploding population, industrialization and increasing urbanization have aggravated the problem (Dak 2002: 1-2). The unemployment, poverty and indebtedness of children's parents are the main causes of child labour in a developing country (Sharma and Mittar 1990: 12). According to ILO, more than 95 per cent of all child workers live in the developing countries. As the world's most populous region, Asia accounts for more than 50 per cent of child labourers. However, Africa has the highest percentage of children working, roughly one in three. In Latin America, an estimated 15 to 20 per cent of all children work (Bhargava 2003: 2). Many jobs that children do are harmful for their health. The manner of their employment, the nature of their work and the contribution under which they are often employed subject them to severe health and safety hazards. Work in agriculture is also characterized by certain hazards, particularly with the introduction of advanced farming practices, new techniques and chemicals. This is also prolonged exposure to heat, sunlight, dust, wind and insects and the high costs in terms of safety and health associated with work in commercial and plantation agriculture. Children are particularly at risk from epidemic and parasitic diseases, diseases of the respiratory tract, dermatosis and fatal accidents. However, these problems are multiplied several fold of industries. Work may be heavy and intense; it may be highly mechanized and extremely monotonous; it may involve the use of sharp and dangerous objects and toxic substances; it may be carried out in conditions of extreme heat, dust and noise.

A World Health Organization report on child workers cites health hazards such as bony lesions and postural deformity attributable to such work as carpet weaving, embroidery and lifting heavy weights. Children generally work for long hours, which results in excessive fatigue and stunted growth. Poor children are generally malnourished but their work increases their energy requirements and calorie deficit. Moreover, if they suffer from anaemia, fatigue and inadequate sleep, they become more susceptible to accidents and infectious diseases. Excessively hot, damp or dusty conditions also create a milieu which favours the transmission of communicable diseases. Many of these diseases, for example, tuberculosis, may be very difficult to cure and involve lifelong illnesses (Gomango 2001: 147-148). Due to working involvement from an early age they are deprived of all the facilities like opportunities for education, leisure and recreation, intellectual development, freedom from exploitation that a society normally offers to its members. Their growing bodies suffer continually from fatigue, overexertion, lack of hygiene and all other problems with which they are confronted. This considerably hinders their harmonious physical and mental development (Panigrahi 2003: 37). Almost all of these activities of children either directly deprive the child from opportunities for full physical and mental development or indirectly cause low level equilibrium in terms of a life-time chance. In fact, sometimes children work in such conditions where would lead to physical handicaps and even cause death. Even when alive, they end up as a family and social burden. It is these consequences which are at the back for once mind when one looks at the social concern for the children which is voiced all-over the world (Chandra 1997: 36-37). Children are gifts of God. They are the blooming flowers of the garden of society. It is, therefore, a duty on the part of each member of society to protect those flowers from each and every kind of damaging effect (Ahmad 2004: 17). It is said that the present child would be the future representative of a society. In this context child health is a very crucial issue for the progress of future society (Biswas and Gan 2008: 52). However, the present study mainly highlights the health profile of working children in the stone crushing sector at Balasan river basin of Darjeeling district, West Bengal.

Methodology

The area was selected on the basis of pilot survey and observation. The village, namely Purba Rangia was selected which was located on Balasan river basin adjacent to Siliguri town under Matigara block, Darjeeling district, West Bengal. Most of the people of this village were engaged in stone based occupation for their livelihood. They earned a very little which was not adequate for eking out a living, so due to poor income the children had to assist their parents financially and that's why this area was selected for the present study. In this regard, the population of 5-14 years age group was taken as child population. Total 50 child workers' families those who were involved with stone crushing job were taken. The findings are based on primary as well as secondary data. Primary data were collected through intensive interviews, case studies, observation, group discussion and preliminary census schedule.

The Studied Families: All of the studied families in this area were migrants. Due to some unavoidable circumstances they were coerced to leave their early place of residence, land and property. As a consequence, they became homeless, landless as well as resourceless. Basically they came here with an empty hand and accepted the stone based occupation as their prime source of income for eking out a living. The studied village was located on Balasan river basin. This river flows downward from Himalaya with natural resources like sands, stones and boulders those are supplied to the outside mainly for building and road construction that's why the stone based occupation is the prime source of income in the studied area. They were migrated here primarily to be involved with such type of occupation in spite of getting little remuneration because they had no sufficient money to invest in any other suitable business or occupation. Thus, seeing no other means, they had to attach with stone based occupation which was the only way of making their living. In the studied families an important highlighting issue is that their little earnings from stone based work did not allow them to lead a normal life with providing the minimum adequate basic necessary livelihood requirements. Hence they needed a monetary support and in many cases the involvement of their children into work was the best solution to get rid of the extreme poverty. Generally they

Table 10.1: Distribution of Child Workers on the basis of Age and Sex

Age group	*No. of child worker*		
	Male	*Female*	*Total*
5-6	4 50.00	4 50.00	8 100.00
7-8	6 42.86	8 57.14	14 100.00
9-10	8 44.44	10 55.56	18 100.00
11-12	10 55.56	8 44.44	18 100.00
13-14	9 52.94	8 47.06	17 100.00
Total	37 49.33	38 50.67	75 100.00

Table 10.2: Distribution of Child Workers' Family on the Basis of Monthly Income (including the Income of Working Children)

Child workers' family	*Monthly Income (in Rupees)*					
	Up to 1000	*1001-2000*	*2001-3000*	*3001-4000*	*4001 and above*	*Total*
No. of family	1 2.00	23 46.00	21 42.00	4 8.00	1 2.00	50 100.00

got involved with various types of stone based activities viz. stone collection and crushing, sand gathering and truck loading.

Health Profile of Working Children

***Working Condition*:** In the studied area most of the children were forced to do the stone based work for an average six to seven hours in a day and even sometimes more than that primarily for mere subsistence which indicated their busy working schedule during day time. The data reveals that 40 per cent, 33.33 per cent and 12 per cent of them used to do this work for 5 to 6 hours, 7 to 8 hours and above 8 hours at a stretch respectively (Table 10.3). Hence they hardly got adequate rest and sleep mainly for their working involvement. In the stone field it was common to observe that during stone crushing work often they made themselves injured either with stone chips or with iron implements which could mostly be seen on their hands, legs and eyes. The data in respect of physical injuries manifests that 18.37 per cent and 18 per cent of the total ailments found in male and female working

Table 10.3: Distribution of Child Workers on the basis of Working Hours in a Day

Child Worker	*Working hours in a Day*					
	1-2	*3-4*	*5-6*	*7-8*	*8+*	*Total*
Male	1 2.70	5 13.51	14 37.84	11 29.73	6 16.22	37 100.00
Female	1 2.63	4 10.53	16 42.11	14 36.84	3 7.89	38 100.00
Total	**2** **2.67**	**9** **12.00**	**30** **40.00**	**25** **33.33**	**9** **12.00**	**75** **100.00**

Table 10.4: Distribution of Male Child Workers on the basis of Type of Diseases

Type of Diseases	*Age Group*					*Total*
	5-6	*7-8*	*9-10*	*11-12*	*13-14*	
Arthritis	—	—	—	—	1 100.00	1 100.00
Dysentery	—	1 9.09	3 27.27	3 27.27	4 36.36	11 100.00
Skin diseases	—	1 11.11	2 22.22	3 33.33	3 33.33	9 100.00
Fever	2 10.00	2 10.00	4 20.00	5 25.00	7 35.00	20 100.00
Jaundice	—	—	—	—	1 100.00	1 100.00
Diarrhoea	—	—	1 25.00	1 25.00	2 50.00	4 100.00
Pneumonia	—	—	—	—	2 100.00	2 100.00
Asthma	—	—	—	—	1 100.00	1 100.00
Total	**2** **4.08**	**4** **8.16**	**10** **20.41**	**12** **24.49**	**21** **42.86**	**49** **100.00**

children respectively (Tables 10.6 and 10.7). But it is a pity that due to their ignorance and negligence of parents the injured eyes often became swelled with burning sensation which created a complex state. Besides this, sometimes minute physical injuries had turned into blisters with mucous secretion just for their improper care of it. In the stone field it was common to notice that at the time of crushing stones the dust

Table 10.5: Distribution of Female Child Workers on the basis of Type of Diseases

Type of Diseases	*Age Group*					*Total*
	5-6	*7-8*	*9-10*	*11-12*	*13-14*	
Arthritis	—	2 20.00	3 30.00	2 20.00	3 30.00	10 100.00
Dysentery	—	1 10.00	2 20.00	4 40.00	3 30.00	10 100.00
Skin diseases	3 13.04	2 8.70	5 21.74	7 30.43	6 26.09	23 100.00
Fever	—	—	—	1 100.00	—	1 100.00
Jaundice	—	—	—	1 33.33	2 66.67	3 100.00
Diarrhoea	—	—	—	—	1 100.00	1 100.00
Pneumonia	—	—	1 100.00	—	—	1 100.00
Asthma	—	—	—	—	1 100.00	1 100.00
Total	**3** **6.00**	**5** **10.00**	**11** **22.00**	**15** **30.00**	**16** **32.00**	**50** **100.00**

emitted out from the broken up stones which was repeatedly being inhaled by them through respiration and as a consequence they might suffer from acute respiratory problem which may have a great probability to turn into chronic asthma in near future when they grow old as it was commonly noticed among the adult and elderly people in the studied area. Due to continuous hard manual labour in a day most of the working children were suffering from various kinds of physical pain found to be common among them which were 28 per cent and 27.55 per cent of the total ailments found in female and male child workers respectively (Tables 10.6 and 10.7). In the stone field it was also observed that a large number of working children had to work for long in touch of river water. Moreover, they had to work under scorching heat of summer, biting cold of winter and under heavy showers and in dusty and polluted environment. Further, the working environment was very much unhygienic and polluted one which might have resulted in numerous health hazards among them throughout the year such as fever, cold and cough, pneumonia, skin diseases, asthma, headache, breathing problem and other minute problems. Thus the working

Table 10.6: Showing Ailments of Male Child Workers

Type of Ailments	*Age Group*					*Total*
	5-6	*7-8*	*9-10*	*11-12*	*13-14*	
Physical injuries	2 11.11	3 16.67	4 22.22	5 27.78	4 22.22	18 100.00
Cold and cough	1 7.14	2 14.29	3 21.43	4 28.57	4 28.57	14 100.00
Physical pain	2 7.41	4 14.81	6 22.22	7 25.93	8 29.63	27 100.00
Headache	—	2 12.50	3 18.75	5 31.25	6 37.50	16 100.00
Teeth and gum problem	—	1 14.29	1 14.29	3 42.86	2 28.57	7 100.00
Malnutrition	1 7.14	1 7.14	3 21.43	5 35.71	4 28.57	14 100.00
Breathing problem	—	—	—	1 50.00	1 50.00	2 100.00
Total	**6 6.12**	**13 13.27**	**20 20.41**	**30 30.61**	**29 29.59**	**98 100.00**

atmosphere indicated an alarming situation which might have leaded to morbid conditions among the working children.

***Food Habit*:** In their daily diet, they mainly took rice with pulses and little amount of vegetables. The feed to the fill was simply unmanageable to most of their parents. Even they could hardly afford eat rice thrice a day. In this respect the quantitative data reveals that a major section of working children (61.33%) could be able to get their meal not more than twice a day (Table 10.10). It was simply beyond the capacity of their parents to cater for milk and other health drinks especially for their children. It can be understood better if we follow the statistical data which manifests that around 80 per cent and 90 per cent of total studied families could hardly accumulate the health drinks and fruits to their children in a year respectively and alongside among the rest percentage it was a seldom happening factor to provide the same as in 16 per cent and 8 per cent of the families it was rarely in a month (Table 10.11). Even they could hardly purchase the least expensive animal protein from the market. The data reveals that 92 per cent and 42 per cent of the studied families were hardly able to accumulate the meat and fishes in a year respectively. On the contrary, only 6 per cent and 48 per cent of the families could manage the least

Table 10.7: Showing Ailments of Female Child Workers

Type of Ailments	Age Group					Total
	5-6	*7-8*	*9-10*	*11-12*	*13-14*	
Physical injuries	2 11.11	3 16.67	5 27.78	4 22.22	4 22.22	18 100.00
Cold and cough	2 12.50	3 18.75	3 18.75	4 25.00	4 25.00	16 100.00
Physical pain	2 7.14	6 21.43	7 25.00	7 25.00	6 21.43	28 100.00
Headache	1 5.88	3 17.65	4 23.53	4 23.53	5 29.41	17 100.00
Teeth and gum problem	—	1 16.67	1 16.67	2 33.33	2 33.33	6 100.00
Malnutrition	1 7.14	2 14.29	3 21.43	4 28.57	4 28.57	14 100.00
Breathing problem	—	—	—	—	1 100.00	1 100.00
Total	**8** **8.00**	**18** **18.00**	**23** **23.00**	**25** **25.00**	**26** **26.00**	**100** **100.00**

Table 10.8: Treatment of Illness of Child Workers

Sex	Type of treatment			
	Traditional	*Quacks*	*Both Traditional and Quacks*	*Total*
Male	5 13.51	1 2.70	31 83.78	37 100.00
Female	4 10.53	1 2.63	33 86.84	38 100.00
Total	**9** **12.0**	**2** **2.67**	**64** **85.33**	**75** **100.00**

expensive animal protein like fishes once in a week and rarely in a month respectively whereas only 8 per cent of the studied families were able to manage the expensive aniinal protein like meat for rarely in a month (Table 10.11). The protein and vitamin deficiencies usually affect the health and its prevalence was noticed among the working children reported from the local quacks also. Indeed, their hard manual work with less nutritive food might have resulted in malnutrition among them which was 14.29 per cent and 14 per cent of the total ailments found in male and female working children respectively. The premature

Table 10.9: Distribution of Child Workers' Family on the Basis of Use of Water

Purpose of Use	*River*	*Well*	*Both Well and River*	*Total*
Drinking	—	11 22.00	39 78.00	50 100.00
Bathing	2 4.00	7 14.00	41 82.00	50 100.00
Household works	1 2.00	17 34.00	32 64.00	50 100.00
Others	4 8.00	17 34.00	29 58.00	50 100.00

Table 10.10: Distribution of Child Workers on the basis of Meal Taken in a Day

Sex	*Meal taken in a day*		
	Twice	*Thrice*	*Total*
Male	20 54.05	17 45.95	37 100.00
Female	26 68.42	12 31.58	38 100.00
Total	**46** **61.33**	**29** **38.67**	**75** **100.00**

entry into work and malnutrition might have an adverse impact on their physical development. Ultimately their utter economic stringency kept them away from nutritious diet required for their heavy workload for day long.

Personal Hygiene: Personal hygiene among the working children in the studied area was serious in condition. A major section of working children in the studied area could never maintain their regular bathing. The use of oil and soap could rarely be seen while bathing. They were likely to be accustomed with taking bath in polluted river water and often in wells. Their unclean bathing may have caused various skin problems. Most of the working children never took regular and proper bath in spite of working in polluted and dusty environment for the whole day. As a consequence, a number of skin problems were often reported among them. The data reveals that the skin diseases were pervasive among them as out of total diseases it was 20 per cent and 18.37 per cent for female and male working children respectively (Tables 10.4 and 10.5). The cleaning of hair regularly and properly was

Table 10.11: Distribution of Child Workers' Family on the basis of Type of Food Taken

Type of food	*Frequency*						
	Daily	*3-4 days in a week*	*1-2 days in a week*	*Once in a week*	*Rarely in a month*	*Hardly accumulate in a year*	*Total*
Rice with minimum amount of vegetables	50 100.00	—	—	—	—	—	50 100.00
Meat	—	—	—	—	4 8.00	46 92.00	50 100.00
Fish	—	—	2 4.00	3 6.00	24 48.00	21 42.00	50 100.00
Egg	—	—	2 4.00	2 4.00	8 16.00	38 76.00	50 100.00
Fruit	—	—	—	1 2.00	4 8.00	45 90.00	50 100.00
Health drinks	—	1 2.00	—	1 2.00	8 16.00	40 80.00	50 100.00

a seldom happening factor while bathing. Ultimately it was almost difficult for the working children to take care of their body cleanliness mainly on account of their prolong working hours a day which always kept them busy and alongside the improper care of parents also responsible for it. Thus in the studied area a major section of working children were not in a position to maintain their good standard of personal hygiene.

***Medical Facilities*:** There was no health centre in the studied area. Therefore, for the treatment of diseases and ailments they had to depend upon both traditional medicine men and quacks. But it was almost impossible to get proper treatment with adequate medicines and necessary diagnostic tests. So, the patients were mostly referred to Matigara Primary Health Centre or North Bengal Medical College only when their condition turned into a critical stage in spite of undergoing a treatment by those local medical practitioners. The proper medical check-up for long time was hardly possible to them primarily due to their severe economic stringency. The data reveals that 85.33 per cent of total studied children had to depend upon both traditional medicine men and quacks as they had no other way to get better treatment (Table 10.8). However, they could not afford to go to the private doctors due to unaffordable expense as they were going through a pernicious pecuniary hardship that's why it was also unbearable for them to expense for proper medical treatment and other required clinical diagnosis. Therefore, the traditional men and quacks of local medicinal shops were their only consultant in respect of treatment which was the only way for them to get rid of for a moment from illness. A large number of parents of working children complained that the Government doctors never paid proper attention and usually neglected them. Among the working children it was generally found that a major section of them were mostly suffering from physical pain through the whole year and it was basically due to their continuous hard physical labour for day long but they paid mere importance on it. In this regard the data reveals that such type of ailments were so pervasive among 28 females and 27 males of the total working children and the percentage against total ailments were 28 per cent and 27.55 per cent of female and male working children respectively (Tables 10.6 and 10.7). In this context their dependency on both traditional medicine men and local quacks for quick remedy was noticed only when it became acute.

Hence, in the studied area most of the working children and their families were debarred of enjoying better medical facilities primarily due to lack of proper medical infrastructure and utter economic stringency. So, to get remedy they had to rely upon the local quacks and traditional medicine men but in many cases their improper treatment of diseases and ailments might have caused a complex situation. Absence of health centre in the studied area was likely to be remained as a great hindrance to develop their health consciousness and awareness as well as they were also dispossessed of getting better treatment with free of cost mainly owing to this fact.

Concluding Remarks

Health is an important part of basic needs for every human being. A healthy child usually indicates a healthy society in future when they grow old because it should be kept in mind that a child is the future representative of a society as well as a nation. However to speak in a word, the health profile of working children including their rest family members in the studied area revealed an unpleasant situation and so many factors were responsible to create such type of ill state like their hazardous working condition, hard physical labour for day long, poor quality and unhygienic food habit, poor standard of personal hygiene, absence of primary health centre, improper care of diseases and ailments, dependency on traditional medicine men and local quacks, lack of health consciousness and awareness, non-accessibility to medical care, poverty and so on. Ultimately such type of hard labourious and venturesome occupation resulted in a number of health hazards among them.

References

Ahmad, A. 2004. *Child Labour in India: A Politico Legal Study*, Delhi: Kalpaz Publications.

Chandra, S.K. 1997. Problems and Issues on Child Labour in India, *Social Change*, 27 (3-4): 34-49.

Bhargava, G. 2003. *Child Labour* Vol. 1, Delhi: Kalpaz Publications.

Biswas, S.K. 2006. Child Worker, Poverty and Hunger: A Study among the Stone Crushers of Balasan River Bed, *Indian Journal of Human Rights and Justice* 2 (1 and 2): 25-37.

Biswas, S.K. and B. Gan 2008. Socio-cultural Factors for Child Survival: A Study on the Resettled Rajbansis of Darjeeling District, West Bengal, *Bulletin of the Department of Anthropology, Dibrugarh University* 36: 43-58.

Dak, T.M. 2002. *Child Labour in India,* Delhi: Serials Publications.

Gomango, S.P. 2001. *Child Labour: A Precarious Future*, Delhi: Author Press.

Panigrahi, M. 2003. Plight of Child Labourers in Rural Orissa, *Indian Anthropologists* 33 (2): 37-51.

Punecha, L.B. 2006. *Child Labour: A Social Evil*, New Delhi: Alfa Publications.

Rizvi, S.N.H. 1991. *Medical Anthropology of the Jaunsaris,* New Delhi: Northern Book Centre.

Sharma, B.K. and V. Mittar 1990. *Child Labour and Urban Informal Sector*, New Delhi: Deep and Deep Publications.

11

Rural Health Care System and Women Health: A Comparative Study on India and Bangladesh

Suchismita Sen Chowdhury

Introduction

"Health system includes all the activities whose primary purpose is to promote, restore or maintain health" (World Health Report 2000). Health care includes preventive, curative and analgesic interventions. The rural health care system aims at providing health services to a large population of the village at the best affordable price. Studies from developed countries demonstrate that an orientation towards a specialist-based system enforces inequity in access. Health systems in low income countries with a strong primary care orientation tend to be more pro-poor, equitable and accessible. At the operational level, the majority of studies comparing services that could be delivered as either primary health care or specialist services show that using primary care reduces physician's costs, and increases patient satisfaction with no adverse effects on quality of care or patient outcomes (Patel 2005). Majority of the rural population in India and Bangladesh are economically backward. Many diseases in rural areas are associated with poverty. Thus, the health system needs to focus on the economic treatment facilities at the rural areas. Since health is not only a physical matter, it also includes mental and social state of an individual. The health care system takes shape according to the need of the population. Thus the system might vary from one country to another. India and Bangladesh are two neighbouring countries having a large population living in the rural areas. About 74 per cent of the India's population lives in rural areas while in Bangladesh 76 per cent of the total population lives in rural areas. It could be find out how the rural health care system has taken shape in these two countries.

In general the women health has been a matter of concern to the social scientist all-over the world. In the Millennium Development Goal (MDG) there were three components associated with health i.e. reducing child mortality, improving maternal health and combating HIV/AIDS, malaria and other diseases. Improving maternal health and reducing child mortality are two important issues in MDG. Women are the most vulnerable group in the rural areas who suffer in silence. Their ill health affects the health of the children. The women bear children and thus they carry forward the human generation. But women's general health needs do not get the necessary attention. There should be special provisions for women in health care services. Now the question is how the two countries have maintained these provisions under rural health care system.

Rural Health Care Infrastructure in India

Primary health care envisages attainment of healthy status for all. Being holistic in nature it is intertwined with diverse principles and components, to provide preventive, promotive, curative and rehabilitative care services. The health care infrastructure in rural areas was developed as a three tier system which included Sub-centre, Primary Health Centre (PHC) and Community Health Centre. Sub-centre was the most peripheral contact point between Primary Health Care System and Community. The population covered under this infrastructure has been shown in Table 11.1.

Table 11.1: Population Covered Under Primary Health Structure in India

Centre	*Population Norm*	
	Plain area	*Hill area/Difficult area*
Sub-centre	5000	3000
Primary Health Centre	30,000	20,000
Community Health Centre	1,20,000	80,000

Source: Rural Health Statistics, MoHFW, GoI, 2007.

Sub-centre (SC): All Primary Health Care Services to the villagers are being provided at the Health Sub-centres. Each Sub-centre has one Female Health Worker/ANM (Auxiliary Nurse Midwife) and one Male Health Worker. One Female Health Assistant (Lady Health Visitor-LHV) and one Male Health Assistant supervise 6 Sub-centres. It plays a vital role in maintaining women health. The activities of the sub-centres are given below:

- The Female Worker takes care of MCH (Mother and Child Health) activities, including Immunization.
- All pregnant women are registered by the Village Health Nurses (VHN) at the earliest stage of pregnancy and given Antenatal care.
- Antenatal care includes two doses of Tetanus Toxied Injections and distribution of 100 tablets of Ferrous Sulphate Tablets (FST).
- Pregnancy complications, if any are referred to higher Medical Institutions like Taluk Hospitals and District Hospitals.
- Deliveries are conducted in Health Sub-centres.
- Village Health nurses provide information on MTP services and are issuing contraceptive tablets, etc. for postponement of next pregnancy.
- Village Health Nurses provide information on sterilization and IUD insertion is done by her.
- The Village Health Nurses guide the local *Dais* and help them in early identification of maternal complicated cases and conduct deliveries under aseptic conditions.
- Male health workers motivate for family planning and distribute condoms.

Rural Health Care System in India 2007

Source: Rural Health Care System in India, 2007

Primary Health Centre (PHC): PHC was a Referral Unit for 6 Sub-centres. The activities of Primary Health Centre involve curative, preventive and Family Welfare Services. A Medical Officer, Block Extension Educator, one female Health Assistant, a compounder, a driver and laboratory technician look after the PHC. At present 14 paramedical and other staff support a Medical Officer. It has 4-6 beds for patients. There are provisions for small surgeries. A PHC covers about 100 villages. A PHC acts as a referral unit for 6 Sub-centres.

The PHCs are established and maintained by the State Governments under the Minimum Needs Programme (MNP)[1] and Basic Minimum Services Programme (BMS)[2]. The Minimum Needs Programme was introduced in the first year of the Fifth Five Year Plan which was thereafter replaced by the Basic Minimum Services in 1996. (*Source*: Planning Commission of India).

The Primary Health Centre deals with—

- Medical care.
- Mother and child health care including family planning.
- Safe water supply and basic sanitation.
- Prevention and control of local diseases.
- Collecting statistical information.
- Health education.
- Training of health guides, health workers, *Dais*.
- Basic laboratory investigations.

Community Health Centre (CHC): Community Health serves as a referral centre for 4 PHCs. CHCs are being established and maintained by the State Government under MNP/BMS Programme. There are four medical specialists i.e. Surgeon, Physician, Gynecologist and Pediatrician supported by 21 paramedical and other staff in a CHC. It has 30 indoor beds with one OT, X-ray, Labour Room and Laboratory facilities. It provides facilities for obstetric care and specialist consultations. Community Health Centre is the largest unit at rural health care infrastructure.

Number of primary health care units has been given in Table 11.2.

Table 11.2: Number of Primary Health Care Units in India

Health Care Unit	*No.*
Sub-centres	1,45,272
Primary Health Centres	22,370
Community Health Centre	4,045

Source: Rural Health Statistics, MoHFW, GoI, 2007.

The number of SCs, PHCs, CHCs are increasing every year. To meet the need of large rural population, the Government of India has taken initiative to set up more PHCs covering more villages. As per the Economic Survey of July, 2009 "There is shortage of 20,855 Sub- centres, 4,833 Primary Health Centres (PHCs) and 2,525 Community Health Centres (CHCs) as per the 2001 population norm", although there has been an improvement in the health sector (Economic Survey 2009).

Rural Health Care Infrastructure in Bangladesh

In Bangladesh public sector health system includes a three tire structure including 5 layers; 3 at primary, 1 at secondary and 1 at tertiary. The structure is as follows:

Primary Level

1. Community clinic and home visitation
2. Union health and family welfare centre
3. *Upazila* health complex

Secondary Level

1. District Hospitals
2. Maternal and Child Welfare Centre (MCWC)

Tertiary Level

1. Health Service Delivery

The health services in Bangladesh are directed by the Ministry of Health and Family Welfare (MoHFW). MoHFW provides most of the HNP (Health, Nutrition, and Population) services. Primary Health Care (PHC) has been chosen by the Government of Bangladesh as the strategy to achieve the goals of "Health for all" which is now being implemented as Revitalized Primary Health Care. The *upazilas* (sub-district) consisting of unions, represent the rural areas of the country. Primary health care service is offered from the union levels called 'Union Health Centres'.

Community Clinic and Home Visitation: With the aim of providing a wide range of health and family planning services through one-stop clinics, capable of delivering an Essential Services Package (ESP) to the vulnerable groups, i.e. women, children, and the poor, the Community Clinics (CCs) were initiated at the grassroot level. Each of these CCs covers an average population of 6,000. The delivery of ESP involves reorganization and restructuring of the existing service-delivery strategies from the existing home-visitation and makeshift outreach facilities (community outlet approach).

Union Health and Family Welfare Centre (UHFWC): At a lower tier Union Health and Family Welfare Centre (UHFWC) are operational, constituted with two or three sub-centres at the lowest administrative level, and a network of field-based functionaries. The public sector field-level personnel are comprised of Health Assistants (HAs) in each union who supposedly make home visits every two months for preventive health care services, and Family Welfare Assistants (FWAs). The FWAs supply condoms and contraceptive pills during home visits. Recently some of the female HAs and FWAs have been trained as birth attendants (skilled birth attendants—SBAs), to provide skilled services within a household. The number of health assistants is determined according to the size of the population. The Health Assistants and Family Welfare Assistants are supervised by a Health Inspector (HI) and a Family Planning Inspector (FPI) respectively, posted at the union level. The UHFWCs provide out-patient care only (WHO 2008).

***Upazila* Health Complex**: *Upazila* health complexes are the first referral system. It comprises of a Medical Assistant and a Family Welfare Visitor. The Medical Assistant has three years of training in disease prevention, health education, and basic first-aid while the Family Welfare Visitor gets 18 months of training in family planning, reproductive health, and post-natal and prenatal care (Perry 2000). These Units have both in- and out-patient services and care facilities. UHCs have in-patient care support with 31 to more than 50 beds. Many UHC Units have a package service called "comprehensive Emergency Obstetric Care services" (EOC) available, with an expert gynaecologist, an anesthetist and skilled support nurses on duty round-the-clock and basic laboratory facilities.

Above the sub-district there are district hospitals (100-250 beds) and medical colleges (serving a group of districts with around 650 beds) providing secondary care, and national tertiary level care facilities. A common tendency is observed in terms of utilization—a stark imbalance in service utilization at public health facilities. There is low utilization of most facilities at the primary level (*Upazila* and below) and over-utilization of facilities at the secondary and tertiary levels. In the Table 11.3, health facilities and services with number of units present in Bangladesh have been depicted.

Table 11.3: Health Facilities and Services in Bangladesh

Facilities	*Services*	*No. in Bangladesh*
Community clinic and home visitation	FP, MCH, immunization, communicable disease control, treatment of common problems and referral.	Not known
Union health and family welfare centre	Out-patient services: Family Planning, Maternal and Child Health, communicable disease control, clinical care, normal delivery and adolescent health care.	4300
Upazila health complex	Out-patient services, impatient services (31-50 beds) with diagnostic and operative treatments	414
District Hospitals	Outdoor and Indoor Services (50-250 beds) with laboratory, radiographic and ambulance services	58
Maternal and Child Welfare Centre (MCWC)	EOC and other related services	55

Source: Ministry of Health and Family Welfare (MoHFW), Bangladesh, 2005.

However, despite such an extensive rural health care infrastructure, only a diminutive fraction, as little as 8 per cent of the rural population accesses these amenities. This 8 per cent is asserted by various NGOs to be made largely for the elite people of the village. Furthermore, of mothers who reported in a household survey that their child was "too sick to eat", only two per cent of them sought care for their child from the nearest Union Health and Family Welfare Centre, most preferring the services of a local village doctor without a medical graduate degree (Perry 2000).

The Women in Rural Health Care System

In the present structural arrangement of the rural health care system and services, maternal and child health has been focused in both the countries. The grassroot level institution of India is the Sub-centre where special assistance is given to the pregnant women and lactating mothers. There is delivery system at the Sub-centre with the trained nurse. The women are informed about birth registration and immunization. In the PHC focus is given on the training of health guides, health workers and *dais* (birth attendant). A Sub-centre covers

5000 people at the plain area. Sterilization is done at the sub-centres. Deliveries are conducted in Health Sub-centres. The immunization for mother and child is also done at Sub-centre. The ICDS centres also monitor the matter in rural areas. Thus these institutions play an important role in women health in rural areas.

The community clinic in Bangladesh focuses on family planning, maternal and child health, immunization, communicable disease control and treatment of common problems. In Bangladesh the success of the immunization depends on the home visits by health workers proximity of outreach clinics (EPI spots and satellite clinics). Many UHC units have a package service called "comprehensive Emergency Obstetric Care services" (EOC) available, with an expert gynecologist, an anaesthetist and skilled support nurses on duty round-the-clock and basic laboratory facilities. In Bangladesh Family Welfare Assistants (FWAs) supply condoms and contraceptive pills. In India the village health nurse takes the initiative to provide information on sterilization and IUD (Intra Uterine Device) insertion. The male health workers distribute condom and motivate the males for family planning.

Health Institutions and the Women

Apart from the health care system in rural areas there are institutions which provide health facilities. For example National Rural Health Mission in India and Health and Population Sector Programme in Bangladesh are two such major institutions which support mother and child health in rural areas.

National Rural Health Mission (NRHM): NRHM (2005-2012) aimed at improving the availability of and access to quality health care by people, especially for those residing in rural areas, the poor, women and children. The goals were—

- Reduction in Infant Mortality Rate (IMR) and Maternal Mortality Ratio (MMR).
- Universal access to public health services such as Women's health, child health, water, sanitation and hygiene, immunization, and nutrition.
- Prevention and control of communicable and non-communicable diseases, including locally endemic diseases.
- Access to integrated comprehensive primary health care.
- Population stabilization, gender and demographic balance.

- Revitalize local health traditions and mainstream AYUSH[3].
- Promotion of healthy lifestyles.

For achieving the goals the capacity of Panchayati Raj Institutions (PRIs) was enhanced, existing PHCs, CHCs and Sub-centres were strengthened (MoHFW 2005).

***Anganwadi* Centre and Integrated Child Development Services (ICDS)**: One *Anganwadi* Centre is sanctioned for 1000 population in rural/urban projects and for 700 populations in tribal projects. *Anganwadi* Centre is managed by an *Anganwadi* Worker, assisted by a *Anganwadi* Helper. Both are honorary workers selected from local community.

ICDS played an important role in the matters of women and child health. ICDS provided package of services, comprising supplementary nutrition, immunization, health check-up, referral services to children below six years of age and expectant and nursing mothers. Another important role it played in educating the women in the age group of 15-45 years regarding health and nutrition. Priority was accorded to the needs of the most vulnerable younger children under three years of age focusing on the capacity building of caregivers to provide stimulation and quality early childhood care.

Nevertheless, there are a number of PHCs, which are successfully delivering service with the help of NGOs.

Health and Population Sector Programme (HPSP): To overcome multidimensional intersectoral problems and to meet the challenges according to the spirit of ICPD[4], Bangladesh Government has launched Health and Population Sector Programme (HPSP) in 1998 in consultation with the development partners and the stakeholders to reform the health and population sector to provide a package of essential health care services to the people and to lower the rate of population growth. HPSP envisioned poverty alleviation with services responsive to client's needs especially those of children, women and the poor and achieve quality of care with adequate service delivery capacity and financial sustainability. The Ministry of Health and Family Welfare and the development partners have worked with a shared vision for achieving objectives of the HPSP.

The main objectives of this programme are:

- Reduction of infant mortality and morbidity.
- Reduction of maternal mortality and morbidity.

- Reduction of fertility.
- Improvement of nutritional status of the people.

These objectives have a specific focus on ensuring access of the disadvantaged groups to high quality client-centred services. Under the present programme the government is implementing Essential Service Package (ESP), which aims to maximize health benefits at a minimum cost, meet felt needs of the clients, strengthen service delivery capacity and improve management system. Within ESP Government's highest priorities are: (a) interventions having public good character, and (b) interventions related to maternal and child health. In line with these priorities the elements of ESP are grouped into five major areas; The ESP covers the following five major areas—Reproductive Health Care, Child Health Care, Communicable Disease Control, Curative Care limited to Basic First Aid, Treatment of Medical and Surgical Emergencies, Pain Relief and Advice, Asthma, Skin Diseases, Eye, Dental and Ear Diseases and at last Behaviour Change Communication (BCC) (ESCAP 2010).

Other aspects

Mother and Child Welfare Centres (MCWC): There are 90 Mother and Child Welfare Centres (MCWC) in the country situated at the District, *Upazila* and Union level which provide antenatal care, normal deliveries, post-natal care; EPI[5], childcare etc.

NGO and Private Sector Services: NGO and private sectors are also involved to provide Reproductive Health services. At present many NGOs have special programme and facilities for providing antenatal care and safe delivery care.

Satellite Clinics: Every month about 30,000 "satellite clinics" are organized at ward and community levels in all-over the country to aim at bring the service facility at the door step of the people to deliver antenatal care, Family Planning, health education and EPI[5] services.

The health institutions actually work in collaboration with the main Government health infrastructure of the respective countries. These institutions facilitate better services at the remote areas through the grassroot level health workers. As far as the Non-Governmental Organizations are concerned, it could be observed that they are more active in Bangladesh than in India. On the other hand, the *Anganwadi* centres providing *Integrated Child Development Services* at the villages in

India makes the women and child health secure to some extent. The *Anganwadi* workers are closely associated with the villagers and since they are women in general, the village women feel free to express their problem to them. Thus these institutions have been very helpful in the context of women and child health.

The National Health Policy and the Women

The National Health Policy, **India** 2001 ensured increased access to women to basic health care and committed highest priority to the funding of the identified programmes relating to women's health.

In 2001, the Government policy on health aimed at achieving an acceptable standard of good health of general population. The objectives were strengthening the infrastructure; decentralize health care delivery through *panchayati raj*, setting up national accounting services and to regulate private practice. Persistent incidence of macro and micro nutrient deficiencies, especially among women and children was one of the priority areas in the National Health Policy.

The objectives of the National Health Policy, **Bangladesh** 2001 include many aspects pointing towards rural health system as well as mother and child health. These objectives related to the above issue are—

- to ensure optimum quality, acceptance and availability of primary health care and governmental medical services at the *Upazila* and Union levels.
- to reduce the intensity of malnutrition among people, especially children and mothers and implement effective and integrated programmes for improving nutrition status of all segments of the population.
- to undertake programmes for reducing the rates of child and maternal mortality within the next 5 years and reduce these rates to be acceptable level.
- to adopt satisfactory measures for ensuring improved maternal and child health at the union level and install facilities for safe and clean child delivery in each village and to improve overall reproductive health resources and services.
- to ensure the presence of full-time doctors, nurses and other officers/staff, provide and maintain necessary equipment and supplies at each of the *Upazila* Health Complexes and Union Health and Family Welfare Centres.

- to strengthen and expedite the family planning programme with the objective of attaining the target of Replacement Level of Fertility and to explore ways to make the family planning programme more acceptable, easily available and effective among the extremely poor and low-income communities.

Mother and Child Health Scenario

Rural women in Asia are among the most disadvantaged people in the world in terms of their health status and access to accurate and appropriate health information and comprehensive, adequate and affordable health services. Sexual and reproductive health is a particular concern for rural women, as a host of social, cultural, political, and economic factors increase Asian rural women's vulnerabilities to pregnancy-and childbirth-related deaths and disabilities, unsafe abortion, HIV/AIDS, and reproductive cancers (Patel, 2005).

The concept of healthy mother and healthy baby is an important aspect of reproductive health care programme. In developing countries like India and Bangladesh, poverty, illiteracy and multiple pregnancies take their toll of mother's health and that of the breast-fed infant. High prevalence of anemia and malnutrition among the reproductive age group women, particularly during pregnancy and lactation can have irrevocable effects on the infant's health.

Table 11.4a and Table 11.4b show the basic health indicators in India and Bangladesh respectively[6].

If these two tables are compared, it will show that the maternal mortality rate was little higher in Bangladesh (1 in 51) than in India (1 in 70). Maternal mortality ratio was very close in two countries. Even in contraceptive prevalence and life expectancy of females as a per cent of males showed hardly any difference. Total fertility rate was more in Bangladesh (3.1) than in India (2.7). Annual number of births per thousand women was much higher in Bangladesh than in India. Life expectancy at birth (years) and Infant mortality rate (under 1) was similar in both the countries, while Under-5 mortality rate was higher in Bangladesh.

The Picture in India

India is facing with an unparalleled child survival and health challenge. Nearly 26 million infants are born each year, of whom 1.2 million die

Table 11.4a: Basic Health Indicators for Women and Children in India

Indicators	*Number/Rate/Ratio*
Maternal mortality rate	1 in 70
Maternal mortality ratio, adjusted (2005)	450
Maternal mortality ratio, Lifetime risk of maternal death. 1 in (2005)	70
Life expectancy: females as a per cent of males	105
Contraceptive prevalence (%), (2003-2008)	56
Antenatal care coverage (%), (2003-2008)	74
Total Fertility rate (per women)	2.7
Annual no. of births (thousands)	26913
Life expectancy at birth (years)	64
Infant mortality rate (under 1)	52
Under-5 mortality rate	69
Neonatal mortality rate, 2004	39
Percentage of infants with low birth weight (2003-2008)	28

Source: UNICEF, 2008.

Table 11.4b: Basic Health Indicators for Women and Children in Bangladesh

Indicators	*Number/Rate/Ratio*
Maternal mortality rate	1 in 51
Maternal mortality ratio, adjusted (2000)	380
Maternal mortality ratio, Lifetime risk of maternal death. 1 in: (2000)	59
Life expectancy: females as a per cent of males	103
Contraceptive prevalence (%), (1997-2005)	58
Antenatal care coverage (%), (1997-2005)	49
Total Fertility rate (per women)	3.1
Annual no. of births (thousands)	3747
Life expectancy at birth (years)	64
Infant mortality rate (under 1)	54
Under-5 mortality rate	73
Neonatal mortality rate, 2000	36
Percentage of infants with low birth weight (1998-2005)	36

Source: UNICEF, 2005.

before completion the first 4 weeks of life and 1.7 million die before reaching the first birthday. WHO/UNICEF addresses the most common conditions responsible for child mortality and morbidity. These include acute respiratory infections (pneumonia), diarrhoea, measles, malaria and malnutrition. The high prevalence of malnutrition contributes to over 50 per cent of child deaths. In India, a significant proportion of child deaths (over 40% of under-five Mortality and 64%

of infant mortality) take place in the neonatal period. Apart from infections, other causes like asphyxia, hypothermia and pre-maturity are responsible for neonatal mortality. About one-third of the newborns have a birth weight less than 2500 gram (low-birth weight). A significant proportion of mortality occurs in low-birth weight babies. It has been recognized that further reduction of IMR will require focused attention on Neonatal mortality (WHO 2009).

WHO has been an active partner of the government in adapting the generic materials suited to meet the needs of the child health programme in India. The adaptation gives due emphasis to management of the neonatal period and supporting mothers and families of newborn babies through domiciliary visits.

The health of the mother and the care she receives during pregnancy, child-birth and the period immediately after birth is inextricably linked with the health of the baby. A critical factor in the continuum of care necessary for favourable maternal and infant outcome is skilled birth attendance. To assist the government in its efforts towards improving skilled birth attendance, WHO is providing assistance in developing Community Level Skilled Birth Attendants.

The Picture in Bangladesh

Maternal mortality and morbidity is a serious concern in Bangladesh. Within the current maternal mortality ratio of 4.0 per 1000 live births, around 16,000 mothers die each year due to causes related to pregnancy and childbirth. It is estimated that complications develop in about 6,00,000 pregnancies of the 4 million women who become pregnant every year. In Bangladesh there are about 9 million women who have survived the rigours of pregnancy and childbirth and suffer from lasting complications. According to the most recent Demographic and Health Survey only 8 per cent of all deliveries are conducted with health facilities.

According to the WHO composite index for overall health system attainment of 191 member states, Bangladesh is ranked 131, worse than India. Two-thirds of the births do not receive any antenatal care. Among those who receive antenatal care, only 16 per cent are informed of the signs of complications, and slightly more than one-third receive iron tablets. For delivery, only 6 per cent use health facilities. Trained health personnel assist deliveries of only 22 per cent of the births.

The complete coverage of immunization is not achieved for almost 50 per cent of the children. Prevalence of acute respiratory infection

(ARI) is high (18.3%) but treatment is sought for only one-fourth of the ARI patients.

Malnutrition continues to be a severe health problem among both mothers and children in Bangladesh. The extent of stunting and underweight are 45 per cent and 48 per cent respectively for children under five years of age, while anemia is prevalent among 53 per cent of pregnant women.

The major causes of death are pneumonia, respiratory failure, injuries, upper respiratory tract infection and diarrhoea, while the major causes of morbidity appear to be ulcer, diarrhoea, malaria, asthma and rheumatism/rheumatic fever (*CPD Task Force Report 2001*).

This sort of health situation is not only the result of economic backwardness of the rural people in these developing countries, but also inadequate structural arrangement of rural health care system. The communication gap between the service providers and the service receivers is another problem in rural areas. The gender dimension in this regard could not be ignored as the women prefer lady doctors instead of male doctors for discussing their problems. But there is hardly any female doctor in the village. So the problem is very much social as well as infrastructural.

Problems in the Healthcare System

India

In India it was found that 21,854 PHCs are established against the 23,100 requirements ideally. The established PHCs face a number of problems, which include staffing, basic amenities, and equipment. Unable to meet the demand hence compliance level is low and they have no monitoring process. India faces a huge need gap in terms of availability of number of hospital beds per 1000 population and non-availability of doctors at emergency. Only 42 per cent of births in the country are supervised by health professionals. Most women deliver with help from women in the family who often lack the skills and resources to save the mother's life if it is in danger. According to UNDP Human Development Report (1997), 88 per cent of pregnant women (age 15-49) were found to be suffering from anemia.

The problem in health care system in the rural areas could be generalized as follows:

1. Inappropriate health policy and infrastructure for rural areas.
2. Inequality in health services in rural areas.

3. Inadequate public health expenditure and misallocation of public money, inadequate funding.
4. There is no system of providing incentives to the private medical practitioners so that they may took interest for working in rural areas.
5. *Growing commercialization of health*—The disillusionment and frustration with the growing ineffectiveness of the government sector is gradually driving poor people to seek help of the private sector, thus forcing them to spend huge sums of money on credit, or they are left to the mercy of 'quacks'.
6. Applying current norms to the population projected for the year 2000, it is estimated that the shortfall in the number of SCs/PHCs/CHCs is of the order of 16 per cent. (Patil *et al.*, 2002).

Bangladesh

It is noted that the highest number of problems (22%) in health sector are related to inadequate number of physicians, wrong treatment, negligence towards patients, absence from duty and unwillingness of doctors to stay at rural areas and small towns. The other problems are related to supplies, equipment, beds etc. (21%). Some other major problems often discussed also include lack of ambulance services as well as proper referral services.

Deficiencies particularly in the rural healthcare centres are:

1. Lack of proper diagnostic facilities
2. Lack of qualified physicians
3. Improper distribution of diagnostic professionals
4. Professional isolation of physicians
5. Medical manpower shortage
6. Post-disastrous medical management

(*Source*: TSLab 2010).

Government complexes are not utilized to "anywhere near their capacity", primarily because of the lack of quality care and accessibility. Alarmingly, less than 50 per cent of the women are even aware of the existence of Satellite Clinics in their areas. According to a national survey undertaken by USAID on disadvantaged Bangladeshis, not even one per cent of those surveyed had utilized the services of a Union Health and Family Welfare Centre (Perry 2000).

Conclusion

Health care covers not merely medical care but also all aspects pro-preventive care too. Nor can it be limited to care rendered by or financed out of public expenditure—within the government sector alone but must include incentives and disincentives for self-care and care paid for by private citizens to get over ill health.

It could be stated that the health care system in both the countries are highly structured. The health institutions played an important role in monitoring women health. The needs of women have been focused widely, but the planning could hardly reach the target population. UHFWC of Bangladesh could be compared with India's sub-centre where health workers (both male and female) interact with the villagers regarding planning and mother and child health issues. But in Bangladesh there is facilities for community clinics at grassroot level covering 6000 people whereas one sub-centre in India covers 5000 people in the plains and 3000 people in the hills. UHC in Bangladesh and PHC in India provides the facilities for both in-patients and out-patients, but a UHC have more beds (30-50 beds) compared to the PHC (4-5 beds). Satellite clinics are very effective in Bangladesh. At the same time the NGOs working in the villages has been helpful for bringing changes in the health sector. But still Bangladesh shows high maternal and child mortality rate. High fertility rate and the population pressure on health sector could be a reason for unparallel health situation. Health and Population Sector programme in Bangladesh and NRHM in India aims at reducing child and maternal mortality rate, fertility rate and these also contribute to the women health as a whole. ICDS at the villages take care of the nutritional requirement of the women and children which is lacking in Bangladesh. The policies which focus women health at large remains mostly in pen and paper as it hardly reaches the poor villagers. The gap is always there among the service holders, service providers and the planners in the developing countries like India and Bangladesh.

Under the population programme family planning has given priority, but the methods have not been utilized properly. The health care system needs to be monitored regularly. Uni-purpose workers should be gradually converted into multi-purpose workers with smaller population to take care of. Remote areas, specially the tribal and feudal areas should be taken care with the help of voluntary organizations. There should be a massive effort in health education specially for the women. In order to find out successful approaches to implementation of key programmes of public health, there is a need to do systematic health system research.

Notes

1. The objective Minimum Needs Programme (MNP) was to establish a network of basic services and facilities of social consumption in all the areas up to nationally-accepted norms. The basic needs of the people identified for this programme are Elementary Education, Adult Education, Rural Health, Rural Roads, Rural Electrification, Rural Housing, Environmental Improvement of Urban Slums and Nutrition.
2. The objective of Basic Minimum Services (BMS) is to give impetus on social development and strengthening of infrastructure.
3. AYUSH—Ayurveda, Yoga, Unani, Siddha, Homeopathy—these have been integrated into the national health delivery system.
4. ICPD—International Conference on Population and Development.
5. EPI—Expanded Programme on Immunization is to reduce mortality, morbidity and disability associated with tuberculosis, tetanus, diphtheria, measles, pertussis and poliomyelitis.
6. The UNICEF data of India included the year 2003 to 2008 and the data of Bangladesh included the year 2000 to 2005 in absence of updated data.

References

CPD Task Force Report, 2001, Policy Brief on "Health and Population Sector Policy", Dhaka.

Economic Survey 2009. *Shortage of 28,000 Health Centres in India,* Electronic Document, http://www.thaindian.com/newsportal/health1/, Accessed February 25, 2010.

Bangladesh Gateway 2010. *Health Policy of Bangladesh-2000*, Electronic Document, http://www.bangladeshgateway.org/healthpolicy.php, Accessed April 4, 2010.

TSLab (Telecommunication System Laboratory) 2010. *Health Care in Bangladesh*, Electronic Document, http://www.tslab.ssvl.kth.se/csd/projects/0606/healthcare%20in%20bangladesh.pdf, Accessed April 1, 2010.

Planning Commission of India, *Human and Social Development*, 9th Five Year Plan (Vol. 2), Electronic Document, http://www. planningcommission. nic.in, Accessed October 25, 2009.

National Rural Health Mission (NRHM) (2005-2012) Electronic Document, http://www.mohfw.nic.in, Accessed May 5, 2009.

Patel, N. 2005, *Evaluating the Role of Primary Health Centres in India*, Indian Express Newspapers (Mumbai) Limited Issue dt. 16th to 31st August.

Patil, A.V. with K.V. Somasundaram and R.C. Goyale 2002. Current Health Scenario in Rural India, *Australian Journal of Rural Health* 10: 129-135.

Perry, Henry B. 2000. *Health for all in Bangladesh*, Dhaka: University Press Ltd.

ESCAP (United Nations Economic and Social Commission for Asia and the Pacific) 2010. *Population Programme and Reproductive Health including Family Planning Programme in Bangladesh,* Electronic Document, http:// www.unescap.org, Accessed February 25, 2010.

Ministry of Health and Family Welfare, Government of India. 2007. *Rural Health Care System in India,* Electronic Document, http:// www.mohfw.nic.in/rural, Accessed February 25, 2010.

UNICEF—Bangladesh-Statistics 2005. Electronic Document, http:// www.unicef.org/Bangladesh-Statistics.html, Accessed February 25, 2010.

UNICEF-India-Statistics 2008. Electronic Document, http://www.unicef.org/ India-Statistics.html, Accessed February 25, 2010.

WHO 2009. *Primary Health Care-Indian Scenario*, Electronic Document, http:/ /www.whoindia.org/ Health_System_Development, Accessed February 27, 2010.

WHO 2008. *Health System in Bangladesh*, Electronic Document, http:// www.whoban.org/health_system_bangladesh.html, Accessed February 27, 2010.

World Health Report, 2000. *Health System: Improving Performance*, Geneva: WHO.

PART 2

12

Role of Climate in Anthropometric Variation: A Study Among Central Indian Population

Rajesh K. Gautam, Dipak K. Adak and *Premananda Bharati*

Introduction

Environment plays a great role in shaping the organism all-over the world. Essence of man's history on this earth is the progression of environment on the habitable surfaces of the earth during human's brief life span. The multiplicity of weather events of a locality or an area is called climate (Landsberg 1982). Bergmann's (1847) and Allen's rules highlight that body size and shape vary with varying temperature conditions. More specifically, the larger the ratio of body surface to body volume or weight and the larger the radiative surface to heat-producing mass, the greater the caloric loss by convention or radiation and the greater the skin area for evaporation (and *vice versa*).

Human physiological adaptability to different environmental conditions has been documented by several studies (Schreider 1963, Little and Hochner 1973, Edholm 1978). Other investigations tried to determine whether or not observed variations in human body size and proportions are consistent with the general 'zoological rules'. The findings on a world scale (Schreider 1964, 1975, Roberts 1978) or on a continental scale (Newman 1953, Schreider 1963, Hiernaux 1968, Hiernaux and Froment 1976) show that climatic clines generally agree with the zoological rules for most anthropometric features.

There is an increasing interest among the human biologist in the field of human ecology, especially in relation to the question of how human body adapts itself to the changing environment. The various 'Mendelian population' with different genetic make-up living under different ecological conditions in India, provides an ample opportunity to the anthropologists and human ecologists to study this problem (Malik *et al.*, 1980). In India, Singh *et al.* (1977) found an inverse relationship between average rainfall of an area and the mean stature. Hiernaux (1974, 1977) suggested the association between stature and annual rainfall as biological adaptation. Accordingly, Abe and Tamura (1980) also examined the morphological variations of the head of subjects in 16 areas of Japan by geographic latitude.

Madhya Pradesh is a state situated in the central part of India. It has no coastline and no international frontier. This state lies over a transitional area between the Indo-Gangetic Plain in the north and the Deccan Plateau in the south. Its physiography is characterized by low hills, extensive plateaus, and river valleys. The elevation of Madhya Pradesh ranges from 300 to 3,900 feet (100 to 1,200). In the northern part of the state the land rises generally from south to north, while in the southern part it increases in elevation towards the west. Important ranges include the Vindhya Range and the Kaimur Hills, located in the west and the north, which rise in places to 460; and the Satpura, Mahadeo, and Maikala ranges, in the south, which have elevations of more than 920 meters. The Dhupgarh Peak (1,350), near Pachmarhi in south-central Madhya Pradesh, is the state's highest point. North-west of the Vindhya Range is the Malwa Plateau (460 to 610). Other features are the Bundelkhand; Plateau, north of the Vindhyas; the Madhya Bharat Plateau, in the extreme north-west; and the Baghelkhand Plateau, in the north-east.

Madhya Pradesh has a sub-tropical climate. Like most of north Indian states it has a hot dry summer (April-June) followed by monsoon rains (July-September) and a cool and relatively dry winter. The average rainfall is about 1,370 mm (53.9 in). It decreases from east to west. The south-eastern districts have the heaviest rainfall, some places receiving as much as 2,150 mm (84.6 in), while the western and north-western districts receive 1,000 mm (39.4 in) or less.

The present study examines the climatic and anthropometric data among the population of 28 districts of Madhya Pradesh to find out if there exists any association between morphology and climate.

Material and Methods

The study sample is based on the basic anthropometric data collected on adult males aged 18-70 years by the Anthropological Survey of India (Basu *et al.* 1994). For present investigation a total of 8441 individuals of 28 districts of Madhya Pradesh were included in the study. The data were collected by the trained physical anthropologists of Anthropological Survey of India. Therefore, it can be well assumed that accuracy of the data is properly taken care of. For convenience, measurements were taken only on adult males who looked apparently normal. Efforts were also made to exclude closely related individuals like brothers and fathers and sons and those with any kind of physical deformities. Therefore, the samples were free from any selection bias.

The data on climate was collected by meteorological stations. Rainfall amount is cumulative rainfall for the past 24 hours measured at 0830 IST of the day. Relative humidity values are calculated as an average of value measured at 0830 and 1730 hours IST. Mean temperature is the average of maximum and minimum temperatures. In this way the data on rainfall, relative humidity and temperature are gathered daily at different meteorological stations all-over the country. On the basis of this daily data of 50 years for rainfall and 30 years of data for rest two factors the district-wise daily were prepared by meteorological data centre Pune. The Average values of climatic factors are drawn for a day from the above data. The data on rainfall was based on from the data collected during 1941-1990; whereas data on temperature and humidity were based on the data collected during 1971-2000.

Results and Discussion

District-wise mean and standard deviation values of eight anthropometric characteristics: stature, sitting height, weight, head length, head breadth, nasal height, nasal breadth and head circumference are presented in Table 12.1. It reveals that the inhabitants of district Ratlam are tallest with an average height of 1668.1 mm and inhabitants of Sidhi district are shortest with mean stature of 1621.0 mm The one-way analysis of variance (ANOVA) shows that the inter-district variation in stature is statistically insignificant as the *F*-ratio is less (*F* ratio = 1.2, $p > 0{\cdot}05$) and insignificant.

The residents of different districts of central India are found to vary in the length of trunk as the mean sitting height is found highest for people of Guna district (842.9±34.9) and shortest for the people of Ujjain district (801.9± 48.2). To find out the inter-district variation one-way analysis of variance (ANOVA) computed, which shows that the variation is significant (*F* ratio = 4.6, p < 0·001). Similarly inter-district variation in mean weight (kg) of central Indian population was found significant (*F* ratio = 2.1, p < 0·001). People of Gwalior are heaviest with mean weight of 53.1 kg. whereas the residents of Ujjain are comparatively lighter in weight with mean weight of 48.4 kg. The measurements taken on head and nose like head length, head breadth, head circumference, nasal height and nasal breadth also show inter-district variation with significant *F* ratio as evident from Table 12.1.

District-wise mean and standard deviation of climatic factors and four anthropometric indices are furnished in Table 12.2. As evident all the indices are showing inter-district variation. *F* ratio value is significant. Similarly, the climatic factors also vary significantly among the districts. Keeping anthropometric variables as dependent and climatic factors as independent, the relationship between biological variables and climatic factors have been studied by Stepwise Multiple Regression Analysis (SMRA). The results are presented in Table 12.3, separately for each dependent variable. Further the selection of independent variables by Stepwise Multilinear Regression Analysis (STPRG) is ranked as 1, 2, 3 respectively, as per their selection in the regression equation and are presented in Table 12.4. In this context the lower values of ranking suggest higher association. It is evident from Table 12.4 that rainfall seems to be principal component for stature and head breadth, temperature is principal component for BMI and head length, and humidity is the principal component for body weight. Overall rainfall plays as principal climatic factors behind biological variation.

Finally, it can be said that the intra- and inter-district variation in Madhya Pradesh may be associated with many biological factors. In this context, it can be mentioned that in fact selection operates ultimately on the overall phenotype of the individual, and every component of the environment determines the nature and intensity of the selection. Therefore, environmentally determined adaptability must itself have a genetic basis produced by selection, and this adaptability will interact with the environmentally rigid adaptations (Harrison 1966). The present study indicates that the climatic factors are playing a very important role in regulating the variation in anthropometric characters in different

Table 12.1: District-wise Mean and Standard Deviations of Eight Anthropometric Characteristics among Central Indian Population

S. No.	District	N	Age (Years) (mm)		Stature		Sitting Height (mm)		Weight (in kg)		Head Length (mm)		Head Breadth (mm)		Nasal Height (mm)		Nasal Breadth (mm)		Head Circumference (mm)	
			Mean	*SD*	*Mean*	*SD*	*Mean*	*SD*	*Mean*	*SD*	*Mean*	*SD*	*Mean*	*SD*	*Mean*	*SD*	*Mean*	*SD*	*Mean*	*SD*
1.	Balaghat	300	37.4	11.2	1637.0	58.5	811.2	36.2	51.0	6.8	187.6	7.1	141.4	5.4	48.2	3.5	37.7	2.7	545.6	16.7
2.	Betul	300	34.9	9.2	1648.0	62.8	814.1	37.0	50.0	6.7	187.7	6.1	142.8	5.4	47.3	3.6	37.8	2.6	532.3	16.5
3.	Chhatarpur	305	35.0	10.5	1636.1	60.7	826.3	34.2	49.7	6.4	187.4	6.9	140.6	5.2	48.6	3.9	37.5	2.9	528.2	15.5
4.	Chhindwara	300	37.6	11.3	1641.1	53.2	809.2	34.4	50.1	6.7	186.9	6.5	141.0	5.2	48.1	3.3	38.2	2.6	545.1	17.1
5.	Dewas	299	36.2	10.6	1635.7	53.7	810.5	25.6	49.3	4.9	187.3	5.4	139.3	4.1	49.2	3.4	37.7	3.2	527.8	23.0
6.	Dhar	300	37.4	11.6	1645.7	58.6	820.5	30.9	51.9	6.6	186.9	6.2	139.0	4.6	49.5	3.8	37.3	2.6	524.6	18.4
7.	Guna	313	33.7	10.9	1652.6	59.5	842.9	34.9	49.8	6.6	189.9	6.6	138.3	4.7	49.9	4.4	38.7	3.2	535.2	15.9
8.	Gwalior	300	33.6	12.5	1665.5	64.3	839.9	36.1	53.1	7.8	192.3	6.2	140.4	4.5	50.4	3.8	36.7	3.0	537.7	22.4
9.	Hosangabad	298	35.8	10.4	1647.9	64.1	810.9	36.6	49.2	7.1	187.7	6.7	142.1	5.2	47.4	3.5	37.9	2.2	529.9	17.5
10.	Indore	300	34.6	11.5	1647.0	55.5	827.4	36.5	51.1	7:1	186.1	6.0	138.5	4.9	47.3	3.5	37.0	3.2	532.2	16.6
11.	Jabalpur	303	35.6	11.3	1638.6	63.1	818.6	39.1	51.0	7.5	187.4	6.2	139.9	5.2	49.0	4.0	38.4	2.8	546.8	16.5
12.	Jhabua	300	35.8	10.8	1627.4	65.1	813.8	41.2	49.2	8.3	186.5	7.0	141.1	5.8	49.0	3.6	37.8	2.6	527.8	17.4
13.	Khargone	300	35.3	10.0	1628.1	58.1	807.5	38.0	49.4	7.7	182.1	8.0	139.9	4.8	48.1	3.7	37.6	2.0	527.4	14.5
14.	Mandla	302	36.1	11.4	1632.7	59.6	819.3	33.8	50.0	7.7	187.7	6.3	140.6	5.3	50.5	3.8	37.1	3.1	530.8	15.6
15.	Mandsour	299	36.1	12.6	1639.1	63.8	824.5	41.9	51.3	8.0	186.6	5.8	136.3	4.9	48.6	4.4	37.3	4.2	529.8	23.1
16.	Panna	306	33.6	9.7	1625.7	62.6	819.2	34.9	49.7	6.6	187.7	6.4	141.6	5.7	48.1	3.8	37.1	2.8	527.6	15.7
17.	Raisen	300	37.0	9.8	1644.0	59.1	814.8	34.2	49.9	6.2	188.3	6.2	140.7	4.8	46.7	3.7	38.3	2.5	529.1	18.0
18.	Ratlam	298	33.2	10.9	1668.1	64.2	823.0	47.5	52.5	7.5	189.4	6.5	138.3	5.1	50.2	3.3	38.1	2.6	531.5	14.0
19.	Rewa	299	35.1	11.2	1629.9	65.0	822.7	35.8	51.2	7.3	186.8	7.1	142.2	5.0	49.5	4.0	37.1	3.3	529.4	16.0
20.	Satna	302	32.6	9.8	1624.8	57.6	815.0	33.5	49.9	6.2	187.9	7.1	141.3	5.2	48.3	3.7	37.1	3.0	529.6	16.2
21.	Sagar	350	37.2	10.6	1640.2	56.6	820.2	33.9	51.5	7.5	188.2	6.1	140.2	5.5	48.4	3.5	38.0	2.7	546.0	18.3
22.	Seoni	300	37.1	11.5	1632.9	55.0	808.7	33.2	50.2	6.5	187.1	7.2	140.1	5.3	48.4	3.6	38.1	2.8	545.6	15.6
23.	Shahdol	299	38.1	10.9	1632.8	60.8	830.6	36.7	48.6	6.9	187.9	6.1	139.4	4.9	47.7	3.4	38.9	2.6	542.2	14.5

(Contd.)

(*Contd.*)

S. No.	District	N	Age (Years) (mm)		Stature		Sitting Height (mm)		Weight (in kg)		Head Length (mm)		Head Breadth (mm)		Nasal Height (mm)		Nasal Breadth (mm)		Head Circumference (mm)	
			Mean	*SD*	*Mean*	*SD*	*Mean*	*SD*	*Mean*	*SD*	*Mean*	*SD*	*Mean*	*SD*	*Mean*	*SD*	*Mean*	*SD*	*Mean*	*SD*
24.	Shajapur	301	34.4	11.4	1650.1	66.3	817.8	36.7	51.5	7.0	187.4	6.3	137.6	5.0	49.7	3.5	38.2	2.5	527.9	15.4
25.	Shivpuri	303	34.9	11.4	1654.2	56.6	829.8	35.1	50.4	6.8	190.8	6.9	138.1	5.0	49.9	4.0	37.8	3.0	532.8	16.2
26.	Sidhi	254	37.0	10.9	1621.0	61.7	804.6	48.5	50.1	5.4	186.8	6.4	139.4	5.5	49.8	4.0	37.7	2.8	526.0	33.6
27.	Tikamgarh	311	34.7	10.4	1645.9	63.7	828.6	40.1	48.5	6.2	188.4	6.7	139.3	5.4	49.0	4.4	37.1	2.9	534.1	15.8
28.	Ujjain	299	35.8	11.6	1634.3	56.7	801.9	48.2	48.4	6.5	184.7	5.8	136.5	4.5	47.0	3.5	36.3	2.7	527.2	33.1
	Minimum		32.6		1621		802		48.4		182		136		46.7		36.3		525	
Maximum			38.1		1668		843		53.1		192		143		50.5		38.9		547	
	F Ratio		1.1		1.2		4.6*		2.1*		3.9*		4.3*		2.5*		2.3*		9.2*	

*p>0·001 at df 27 (between group), 8413 (within group) and 8440 (total)

Table 12.2: District-wise Mean and Standard Deviations of Climatic Factors and Anthropometric indices among Central Indian Population

S. No.	District	Rainfall (mm) per day		Temperature (°C) per day		Relative Humidity per day (%)		BMI (kg m^{-2})		Cormic Index		Cephalic Index		Nasal Index	
		Mean	SD	Mean	SD	Mean	SD	Mean	SD	Mean	SD	Mean	SD	Mean	SD
1.	Balaghat	4.0	5.8	24.3	4.7	62.3	18.7	19.0	2.1	0.496	0.016	75.4	3.5	78.6	7.8
2.	Betul	3.0	4.0	24.5	4.3	58.4	19.9	18.4	2.1	0.494	0.018	76.1	3.5	80.2	8.0
3.	Chhatarpur	3.0	4.5	25.9	6.2	57.6	16.8	18.5	1.9	0.505	0.014	75.0	3.6	77.7	8.5
4.	Chhindwara	3.3	4.4	23.9	4.6	61.1	14.6	18.6	2.0	0.493	0.016	75.5	3.3	79.8	7.8
5.	Dewas	2.9	4.3	26.1	4.8	55.5	17.4	18.4	1.6	0.496	0.014	74.4	2.8	76.9	8.3
6.	Dhar	2.3	3.4	26.0	3.2	63.0	10.5	19.1	2.1	0.498	0.015	74.4	3.2	75.7	7.1
7.	Guna	2.9	4.3	25.1	5.6	51.8	19.2	18.2	2.0	0.510	0.014	72.9	3.1	78.0	8.7
8.	Gwalior	2.4	3.5	25.5	6.7	51.6	17.3	19.1	2.2	0.505	0.015	73.1	3.1	73.1	8.8
9.	Hosangabad	3.9	5.9	24.2	4.9	55.5	20.5	18.1	2.3	0.492	0.018	75.8	3.2	80.5	7.3
10.	Indore	2.6	3.7	25.1	4.5	50.5	19.9	18.8	2.3	0.502	0.017	74.5	2.8	78.6	8.2
11.	Jabalpur	3.4	5.0	25.7	5.2	57.7	18.6	19.0	2.3	0.500	0.018	74.7	3.2	79.1	8.6
12.	Jhabua	2.3	3.6	25.9	4.1	52.4	17.8	18.6	2.7	0.500	0.020	75.8	3.5	77.4	6.8
13.	Khargone	2.3	3.2	26.9	4.5	49.8	18.3	18.6	2.6	0.496	0.020	76.7	3.3	78.6	6.7
14.	Mandla	4.0	5.6	24.4	5.0	59.8	18.7	18.7	2.4	0.502	0.015	75.0	3.3	74.1	8.9
15.	Mandsour	2.4	3.7	25.2	4.7	53.8	17.9	19.0	2.5	0.503	0.019	73.1	3.1	75.7	9.1
16.	Panna	3.2	4.9	24.6	5.8	56.7	18.0	18.8	1.9	0.504	0.016	75.5	3.5	77.5	8.8
17.	Raisen	3.4	5.2	24.7	5.7	58.2	17.6	18.4	1.9	0.496	0.018	74.8	3.1	82.4	8.1

(*Contd.*)

(Contd.)

S. No.	District	Rainfall (mm) per day †		Temperature (°C) per day†		Relative Humidity per day (%) †		BMI (kg m-2)		Cormic Index		Cephalic Index		Nasal Index	
		Mean	SD	Mean	SD	Mean	SD	Mean	SD	Mean	SD	Mean	SD	Mean	SD
18.	Ratlam	2.6	3.9	25.7	4.4	54.9	18.4	18.9	2.5	0.492	0.038	73.1	3.3	76.0	6.8
19.	Rewa	3.1	4.5	25.1	5.9	57.0	15.5	19.2	2.0	0.505	0.014	76.2	3.6	75.7	8.3
20.	Satna	3.0	4.2	25.8	5.8	54.5	18.7	18.9	1.9	0.502	0.015	75.3	3.8	77.1	8.8
21.	Sagar	3.3	4.8	25.5	4.8	53.7	20.3	19.1	2.4	0.500	0.016	74.5	3.4	78.7	7.8
22.	Seoni	3.6	4.9	25.6	4.3	55.0	18.3	18.8	2.2	0.496	0.017	74.9	3.7	79.1	8.2
23.	Shahdol	3.4	4.5	24.8	5.4	62.9	15.8	18.2	2.0	0.509	0.015	74.2	3.3	82.0	8.7
24.	Shajapur	2.8	4.3	25.1	5.2	53.6	18.0	18.9	2.2	0.496	0.019	73.5	3.0	77.1	6.6
25.	Shivpuri	2.5	3.7	24.5	5.9	53.4	16.7	18.4	2.0	0.502	0.017	72.4	3.1	76.3	8.7
26.	Sidhi	3.2	4.5	25.8	5.8	57.5	16.6	19.0	1.6	0.496	0.025	74.7	3.5	76.1	8.7
27.	Tikamgarh	2.9	4.5	25.1	5.9	61.1	14.1	17.9	1.9	0.504	0.020	74.0	3.7	76.0	9.4
28.	Ujjain	2.5	3.7	24.6	4.7	56.7	17.6	18.1	2.1	0.491	0.028	74.0	3.0	77.6	7.5
	F Ratio	4.8*		6.6*		15.8*		2.2*		5.4*		2.4*		2.6*	

*$p > 0{\cdot}001$ at df 27 (between group), 10192 (within group) and 10219 (total) for three climatic factors.
For BMI, Cormic, Cephalic and Nasal Index it is at df 27 (between group), 8413 (within group) and 8440 (total).

Table 12.3: Bivariate (linear) and Multivariate Regression between Anthropometric and Climatic Factors among Central Indian Population.

Dependent Variable	*Independent Variables*	*S. No.*	R^2	*B ± SE*	*df*	*F-value*	*t-value*	*P-value*
Stature	Rainfall	R	0.063	-5.7±4.3	27	1.7	-1.3	0.196
	Temperature	T	0.033	-2.9±3.1	27	0.8	-0.9	0.357
	Humidity	H	0.031	-0.6±0.6	27	0.8	-0.9	0.369
	R+T+H		0.208	—	27	2.1	—	0.126
Weight	Rainfall	R	0.039	-0.4±04	27	1.0	-1.0	0.312
	Temperature	T	0.023	0.2±0.3	27	0.6	0.7	0.443
	Humidity	H	0.042	-0.06±0.06	27	1.1	-1.0	0.297
	R+T+H		0.056	—	27	0.4	—	0.704
BMI	Rainfall	R	0.003	0.03±0.1	27	0.07	-0.2	0.788
	Temperature	T	0.094	0.1±0.09	27	2.7	1.6	0.113
	Humidity	H	0.015	-0.01±0.01	27	0.3	-0.6	0.537
	R+T+H		0.109	—	27	0.9	—	0.419
Head Breadth	Rainfall	R	0.261	1.6±0.5	27	9.2	3.0	0.005
	Temperature	T	0.026	-0.3±0.4	27	0.7	-0.8	0.411
	Humidity	H	0.059	0.1±0.08	27	1.6	1.2	0.214
	R+T+H		0.274		27	3.0		0.050
Head Length	Rainfall	R	0.009	0.3±0.6	27	0.2	0.4	0.633
	Temperature	T	0.080	-0.7±0.4	27	2.2	-1.5	0.146
	Humidity	H	0.0	0.007±0.09	27	0.006	0.07	0.939
	R+T+H		0.091		27	0.8		0.505

Table 12.4: Ranking of Climatic Factors in Biological Variables Estimation

Biological factors	*Climatic factors*		
	Rainfall	*Temperature*	*Humidity*
Stature	1	2	3
Weight	2	3	1
BMI	3	1	2
Head Breadth	1	3	2
Head Length	2	1	3
All categories and biological variables combined	9	10	11

districts of Madhya Pradesh. However, it warrants further intensive investigations to find out the various causes of intra- and inter-district population variation in this state, taking into consideration the biological, social and environmental factors.

References

Abe, K. and S. Tamura. 1980. The Ryukyu Islanders and the Inhabitants in South Kyushu of Japan-Morphometric variation by Geographical orders, *In* I.P. Singh and S.C. Tiwari (eds.), *Man and His Environment*, New Delhi: Concept Publishing Company.

Allen, J.A. 1977. The Influence of Physical Conditions in the Genesis of Species, *Radical Review* 1: 108-140.

Basu, A. with D.P. Mukherjee and P.C. Dutta. 1994. *All India Anthropometric Survey: North Zone: Basic Anthropometric Data, Vol. 1. Madhya Pradesh*, Calcutta: Anthropological Survey of India.

Bergmann, C. 1847. Uber die Verhaltnisse der Warmeokonomie des Thiere zuihrer Grosse, *Gottinger Studien* 3:595-708.

Edholm, O.G. 1978. Man—Hot and Cold. *Studies in Biology* No. 97. London: Edward Arnold.

Hiernaux, J. 1968. La diversite humane en Afrique sub-saharienne. Researches biologiques. Bruxells: Editions de I'Institut de Sociologie de I'Universite Librede Bruxelles.

—— 1974. *The People of Africa,* London: Weidenfeld and Nicolson.

—— 1977. Long term effects of Human Migration from the African Savannah to the Equatorial Forests: A Case Study of Human Adaptation to Hot and Wet Climate, *In* G.A. Harrison (ed.), *Population Structure and Human Variation*. IBP No. 11:187-217.

Hiernaux, J. and A. Forment. 1976. The Correlations between Anthropological and Climatic Variables in Sub-Saharan Africa: revised estimates, *Human Biology* 48:747-767.

Landsberg, H.E. 1982. Human Adaptation to Climate, *Mazingira* 6:30-42.

Little, M.A. and D.H. Hochner. 1973. Human Thermoregulation, Growth and Mortality, *An Addison-Wesley Module in Anthropology*, No. 36.

Malik, S.L. with M.K. Bhasin and I.P. Singh 1980. Communities, Caste and Tribes of India: An overview of Morphometric Variation, *In* O.G. Eiben (ed.), *Man and His Environment.*, New Delhi: Concept Publishing Company.

Newman, M. 1953. The Application of Ecological Rules to the Racial Anthropology of the Aboriginal new-world, *American Anthropologist* 55:311-327.

Roberts, D.F. 1978. *Climate and Human Variability* 2nd edition, London: Cummings.

Schreider, E. 1963. Physiological Anthropology and Climate Variations, *In* Environmental Physiology and Psychology in Arid Conditions, Proceedings of the Lucknow Symposium, UNESCO, Paris.

—— 1964. Ecological-Rules, Body-heat Regulation, and Human Evolution, *Evolution* 18:1-9.

—— 1975. Morphological Variations and Climatic differences, *Journal of Human Evolution* 4:529-539.

Singh, I.P. with M.K. Bhasin and S.L. Malik. 1977. Anthropometric Variables in the Indian Population: An Environmental Perspective, *In* O.G. Eiben (ed.), *Growth and Development;* Physique. Symp. Biol. Hung. 20. Akademiai Kiado, Budapest.

13

Assessing Obesity in Adult Bengalee Males in India

Jyoti Ratan Ghosh and *Arup Ratan Bandyopadhyay*

Introduction

Obesity is a condition characterized by an excess of body fat (Low *et al.* 2009). According to the World Health Organization (WHO 2006) there are about 400 million obese adults worldwide in 2005 and by 2015, it will be more than 700 million. The fundamental cause of obesity is an energy imbalance between calories consumed on the one hand, and calories expended on the other hand. A global increase in obesity is attributable to a number of factors including shift in diet towards increased intake of energy-dense foods that are high in fat and sugars but low in vitamins, minerals and other micronutrients; and a trend towards decreased physical activity (WHO 2006). Obesity poses a serious health burden as it is associated with an increased risk of chronic diseases such as diabetes mellitus, cardiovascular disease, musculoskeletal disorders and some forms of cancer (WHO 2006, Razak *et al.* 2007, Low *et al.* 2009). Thus, it is important to develop appropriate anthropometric measure for assessing obesity in order to identify and prevent the development of obesity and related disorders (Yang *et al.* 2007).

The use of anthropometry as an indicator of nutritional and health status of adults is now well established. Body Mass Index (BMI) is a simple index of weight-for-height that is commonly used in classifying obesity in adult populations and individuals. It is defined as the weight in kilograms divided by the square of the height in meters (kg/m^2). Although adult nutritional status can be evaluated in many ways, BMI provides the most useful population-level measure of obesity as it is the same for both sexes and for all ages of adults (WHO 2006). Moreover, it is inexpensive, non-invasive, and suitable for large-scale survey (Bose *et al.* 2006). BMI is generally considered a good indicator of not only the nutritional status but also the socio-economic condition of a population, especially adult populations in developing countries (Bose *et al.* 2006). However, since 1995, there have been several studies, which have attempted to identify an appropriate BMI cut-off value for assessing obesity in adults (WHO 1995, WHO 2000, Ghosh and Bandyopadhyay 2007). The present study was undertaken to assess the obesity, based on different BMI cut-off values, in adult Bengalee males to determine which of these cut-off values was better for assessing obesity.

Materials and Methods

The sample of the present cross-sectional study comprised 180 adult Bengalee men aged 25-67 years, from West Bengal, India. Individuals were informed by letters and oral communication regarding the aims and objectives of the present study. Interested individuals were incorporated and those who were under medication were excluded from the present study. Information on ethnicity, age, occupation and educational status were obtained from all subjects with the help of a questionnaire.

Anthropometric measurements were made by trained investigators using the standard techniques (Lohman *et al.* 1988). Height and weight were measured to the nearest 0.1 cm and 0.5 kg. respectively. Errors of measurements were computed and they were found to be within acceptable limits (Ulijaszek and Kerr 1999). Body Mass Index (BMI) was computed using the following standard equation: BMI (kg/m^2) = Weight (kg)/height (m^2). Per cent Body Fat (PBF) was measured using bioelectrical impedance (OMRON HBF-302).

Obesity was assessed by the followings, internationally accepted WHO's BMI cut-off value (WHO 1995), WHO's proposed BMI cut-off value (WHO 2000) for Asians, total body fat greater than twenty-five per cent (Hortobagyi *et al.*, 1994) and by using the cut-off value proposed for adult Bengalee males (Ghosh and Bandyopadhyay 2007).

The following cut-off values were used for obesity: BMI ≥ 30 kg/m² (WHO, 1995), BMI ≥ 25 kg/m² (WHO 2000), PBF ≥ 25 per cent (Hortobagyi *et al.* 1994) and BMI ≥ 24 kg/m² (Ghosh and Bandyopadhyay 2007). Statistical analysis was performed using the Statistical Package for Social Sciences, version 11.0. (SPSS Inc, Chicago, IL, USA).

Results and Discussion

The mean age of the men was 44.56±9.37 years. The mean and SD of height, weight, PBF and BMI are presented in Table 13.1. Table 13.3 presents the frequency of obesity, based on different BMI cut-off values as well as PBF, among the men. The result (Table 13.3) of the present study revealed that, when PBF (≥ 25%) was used as a gold standard measure of obesity, 100 (55.6%) males were truly obese. However, the results differ when international (≥30.0kg/m²) and proposed (≥25.0kg/m²) cut-off point of BMI were applied for the assessment of obesity (WHO 1995, WHO 2000), seven (3.9%) and sixty-two (34.4%) males were found to be obese. Thus, the cardinal feature was that both international and proposed BMI cut-off values underestimate the prevalence of obesity by 51.7 per cent and 21.2 per cent, respectively. This might be due to the fact that, both international and proposed BMI cut-off values (Table 13.2) have low sensitivity (10.46% and 62.75%, respectively) and comparatively higher specificity (99.64% and 93.50%, respectively) in assessing obesity in adult Bengalee males (Ghosh and Bandyopadhyay 2007).

Table 13.1: Characteristics of the Studied Population

Variables	*Mean*	*Standard Deviation*
Age (year)	44.56	9.37
Height (cm)	164.92	6.35
Weight (kg)	65.33	11.01
Per cent body fat	25.10	4.53
Body mass index (kg/m²)	23.95	3.31

The lower sensitivity as well as higher specificity of international and proposed BMI cut-off points (WHO 1995) might be due to the ethnic variation in the relationship between BMI, percentage of body fat and body fat distribution (WHO 2000). Considering all these facts, in 2000, The International Association for the Study of Obesity (IASO), the International Obesity Task Force (IOTF) and the WHO emphasized on the development of population specific cut-off point for assessing obesity (WHO 2000).

Table 13.2: Sensitivity and Specificity of BMI Cut-off Values to Evaluate Obesity

Cut-off Values	*SN (95% CI)*	*SP (95% CI)*	*OM*
†BMI ≥30kg/m²	10.46% (7.5,13.3)	99.64% (99.0,100)	32.10%
‡BMI ≥25kg/m²	62.75% (58.1,67.3)	93.50% (91.1,95.8)	17.40%
#BMI ≥24kg/m²	83.66% (80.1,87.1)	90.61% (87.8,93.3)	11.80%

From Ghosh JR and AR Bandyopadhyay, 2007, *Coll. Antropol.*, 31:705-708.

†, WHO international cut-off point; ‡, WHO cut-off point proposed in 2000; #, Ghosh and Bandyopadhyay, 2007; SN = Sensitivity; SP = Specificity; OM = Overall misclassification.

Table 13.3: Prevalence of Obesity

BMI Cut-off Values for Assessing Obesity	*n*	*Prevalence of Obesity (%)*
†BMI =30kg/m²	7	3.9
‡BMI =25kg/m²	62	34.4
#BMI =24kg/m²	87	48.3
PBF = 25%	100	55.6

+, WHO international cut-off point; ‡, WHO cut-off point proposed in 2000; #, Ghosh and Bandyopadhyay, 2007.

In the present study, when we used a population specific BMI cut-off value of ≥ 24.0kg/m², 87 males were obese with a prevalence of 48.3 per cent. Which differ by only 7.3 per cent, instead of 51.7 per cent for international cut-off value and 21.2 per cent for proposed cut-off point, from the true prevalence of obesity, measured by gold standard (48.3% vs. 55.6%). Thus, in conclusion, a lower BMI cut-off point of ≥ 24.0kg/m² could be a better option for assessing obesity in adult Bengalee males.

Acknowledgements: Authors are grateful to the all participants.

References

Bose, K. with F. Chakraborty, K. Mitra and S. Bisai 2006. Nutritional Status of Adult Santal Men in Keonjhar District, Orissa, India, *Food Nutr. Bull.* 27:353-356.

Ghosh, J.R. and A.R. Bandyopadhyay 2007. Receiver Operating Characteristic Curve Analysis of BMI in Assessing Obesity among adult Bengalee Males in India, *Coll. Antropol.* 31:705-708.

Hortobagyi, T. with R.G. Israel and K.F. O'Brien 1994. Sensitivity and Specificity of the Quetelet Index to assess Obesity in Men and Women, *Eur. J. Clin. Nutr.* 48:369-375.

Lohman, T.G. with A.F. Roche and R. Martorell 1988. *Anthropometric Standardization Reference Manual,* Chicago: Human Kinetics Books.

Low, S. with M.C. Chin, S. Ma, D. Heng and M. Deurenberg-Yap 2009. Rationale for Redefining Obesity in Asians, *Ann. Acad. Med. Singapore.* 38:66-74.

Razak, F. with S.S. Anand, H. Shannon, V. Vuksan, B. Davis, R. Jacobs, K.K. Teo, M. McQueen and S. Yusuf 2007. Defining Obesity cut points in a Multiethnic Population, *Circulation.* 115:2111-2118.

Ulijaszek, S.J. and D.A. Kerr 1999. Anthropometric Measurement Error and the Assessment of Nutritional Status, *Br. J. Nutr.* 82: 165-177.

WHO/IASO/IOTF 2000. *The Asia-Pacific Perspective: Redefining Obesity and Its Treatment*, Melbourne: Health Communications Australia.

World Health Organization 2006. *Fact sheet: Obesity and Overweight,* Electronic document, http://www.who.int/mediacentre/factsheets/fs311/en/print.html. Accessed March 21, 2010.

World Health Organization 1995. *Physical Status: the Use and Interpretation of Anthropometry*, Technical Report Series no. 854, Geneva.

Yang, J.J. with K. Shiwaku, T. Nabika, J. Masuda and S. Kobayashi 2007. High Frequency of Cardiovascular Risk Factors in Overweight Adult Japanese Subjects. *Arch. Med. Res.* 38:337-344.

14

Metabolic Syndrome in a Peri-Urban Population: The Paundra Kshatriya of South 24-Parganas, West Bengal

N.K. Bagchi and *D.K. Adak*

Introduction

The 'Metabolic Syndrome', a group of risk factors associated with development of cardiovascular disease and Type 2 diabetes, has reached epidemic proportions in western societies and has emerged as a major public health problem. The hallmark of the syndrome is a co-occurrence of obesity, dyslipidemia, carbohydrate intolerance and hypertension. With insulin resistance as the common denominator, it is also referred to as the "insulin resistance syndrome". However, the role of insulin resistance as the central feature of the syndrome, particularly of its association with cardiovascular diseases remains uncertain. In 1998, WHO proposed a unifying definition for the syndrome and chose to call it the 'metabolic syndrome' rather than the 'insulin resistance syndrome' (Alberti and Zinmet 1998).

A tangible concept of the syndrome was, however, first provided in the Banting lecture by Reaven (Reaven 1988), which he called the syndrome X, and suggested that insulin resistance is associated with a series of metabolic risk factors for cardiovascular diseases. The syndrome has been given several names, including the 'metabolic syndrome', the 'insulin resistance syndrome', the 'plurimetabolic syndrome', and the 'deadly quartet'. The mechanisms underlying the metabolic syndrome are not fully known, however, resistance to insulin stimulated glucose uptake seems to modify biochemical responses in a way that predisposes to metabolic risk factors (Gogia and Agarwal 2006). The Third Report of the National Cholesterol Education Programme (NCEP) Adult Treatment Panel (ATP III) included clinical diagnosis guidelines for the Metabolic Syndrome. Compared with findings from earlier studies and WHO guidelines the new ATP III defines criteria measured in clinical practice (Vega 2001).

The clinical relevance of the metabolic syndrome is related to its role in the development of cardiovascular disease. The incidence of coronary disease along with carotid atherosclerosis is higher in patients with metabolic syndrome along with higher mortality from all such causes (Haffner *et al.* 1986).

Approximately one-fourth of the US adults 20 years or older meet the diagnostic criteria for metabolic syndrome. The prevalence of the metabolic syndrome depends on age, ethnic background, and gender. It rises linearly from 20 to 50 years and plateaus thereafter. Looking at various studies around the world, which included population samples, aged from 20 to 25 and upwards, the prevalence varies from 8 per cent (India) to 24 per cent (United States) in men and from 7 per cent (France) to 46 per cent (India) in women.

In line with the rising prevalence of obesity, the metabolic syndrome is also increasing in developing countries. The prevalence of insulin resistance in Asian Indians residing in India ranged from 20 to 55 per cent, the prevalence was due to heterogeneity of the population (higher in urban than rural) and socio-economic strata (SES). The prevalence is higher in the people belonging to high SES in comparison with low SES (Misra *et al.* 2002, Wasir and Misra 2004). Two Indian studies, both are on population based sample within the age range but reported prevalence of 13 per cent in Jaipur and 41 per cent in Chennai (Gogia and Agarwal 2006). A third Indian study, also from Chennai, reported a metabolic syndrome prevalence of 11.2 per cent, which was much closer to the prevalence rate reported for Jaipur. However, within the same ethnic population group there can be significant differences in the prevalence of metabolic syndrome (Gogia and Agarwal 2006). Metabolic syndrome prevalence varies among ethnic groups. In this study we examine the prevalence of metabolic syndrome in a peri-urban population namely Paundra Kshatriya of South 24-Parganas district, West Bengal.

Materials and Methods

The area of present study, namely Sonarpur, South 24-Parganas, West Bengal is well connected with roads to the city centre, Kolkata. The Poundra Kshatriya or Pod (caste) forms the largest segment of the heterogeneous population in the study area. They are considered as the disadvantaged population in terms of overall socio-economic development. The community is a combination of landowning and landless people. Only a few families can fully maintain themselves with earnings from their land (Singh 2008). Poundra Kshatriya residing in this region is largely dependent on various kinds of occupation for their subsistence economy. The males are mainly engaged in self-employment (33.85%) and different types of white collar job (27.43%). A good number of them are also engaged in skilled (17.95%) and non-skilled (13.85%) jobs. The females are engaged in non-skilled (4.27%), skilled (2.40%), white collar job (3.73%) and self-employment (2.93%) service in a very low frequency. However, as expected, majority of the females in this population group are found to be engaged as housewife (86.13%).

For the purpose of present study data were collected from unrelated adult individuals (males and females) belong to the Poundra Kshatriya community. Altogether 98 males and 142 females were considered for the sake of present study. On the basis of these samples two categories were made—(i) Normal: subjects without any symptom of metabolic syndrome and (ii) M.S.: subjects with metabolic syndrome. Among the males 60 subjects are identified as normal and the rest i.e. 38 are having metabolic syndrome, whereas among the females 108 subjects are normal and 34 are having metabolic syndrome.

Data on anthropometry and arterial pressure were collected while the respective households were visited. Side by side, blood samples were collected from the unrelated individuals who were on 12 hour fasting. The blood samples were transported soon after collection and analyzed in the laboratory of Anthropological Survey of India, Kolkata. The analysis is done with the help of Semi Auto Analyzer, Minitechno, derived by Logotech India Pvt. Ltd.

Two definitions of metabolic syndrome have been adopted in most studies: (i) proposed by the World Health Organization (WHO) and (ii) Third Report of the National Cholesterol Education Programme (NCEP) Adult Treatment Panel III (ATP III).

In the present study the definition of NCEP has been followed. The definition of NCEP does not explicitly include insulin resistance or glucose intolerance as required criteria, rather defines the syndrome as the co-occurrence of three or more of the following five criteria:

- Abdominal obesity—waist circumference >102 cm in men and >88 cm in women;
- Triglycerides >150 mg/dL;
- HDL cholesterol <40 mg/dL in men and <50 mg/dL in women;
- High blood pressure >130/85 mm Hg;
- Fasting plasma glucose >110mg/dL.

We have followed a working definition as proposed in ATP III with the exception that we have used BMI (>25 kg/m^2) and or WHR (>0.90) as predictors of obesity.

Results

Descriptive statistics of the traits related to metabolic syndrome are presented in Table 14.1, while in Figure 14.1 the results are shown graphically. Mean age of the studied males and females are 47.17 and 38.44 respectively. Systolic and diastolic blood pressure in general is in normal level in this population. All other traits are at higher level than the normal range in this population. Waist-hip ratio (male: 0.9307;

Table 14.1: Descriptive Statistics of the Examined Traits

Traits	*Male (n = 98)*			*Female (n = 142)*			*t-value*
	Mean	*S.D.*	*S.E.*	*Mean*	*S.D.*	*S.E.*	
Age (years)	47.17	14.46	1.46	38.44	11.88	1.00	4.93**
BMI (kg/m^2)	23.07	3.51	0.35	24.14	4.11	0.34	2.18*
WHR	0.9307	0.07	0.01	0.8734	0.09	0.01	4.09**
SBP	126.52	22.12	2.23	128.80	21.00	1.76	0.80
DBP	80.37	11.87	1.20	83.62	12.83	1.08	2.02*
TG (mg/dl)	131.57	41.23	4.16	124.39	42.29	3.55	1.31
FPG (mg/dl)	99.41	23.01	2.32	94.06	16.98	1.42	1.97*
HDL (mg/dl)	42.88	11.45	1.16	48.42	13.18	1.11	3.46**

BMI = body mass index; WHR = waist-hip ratio; SBP = systolic blood pressure; DBP = diastolic blood pressure; TG = triglyceride; FPG = fasting plasma glucose; HDL = high = density lipoprotein cholesterol

★ Significant at 0.05 level of probability.

★★ Significant at 0.001 level of probability.

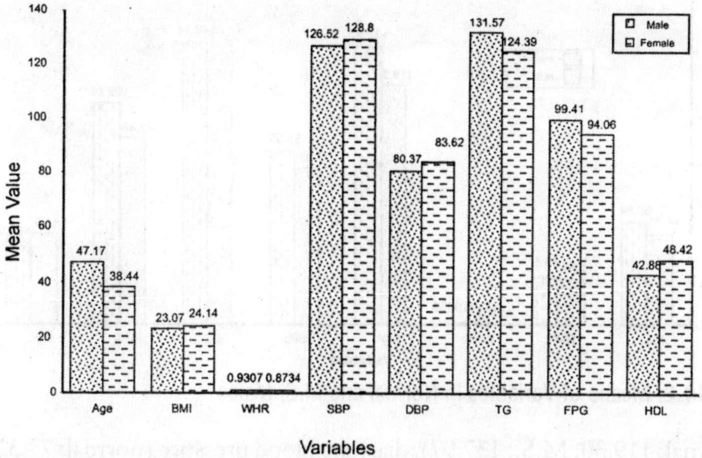

Fig. 14.1: Means of Different Variables

female: 0.8734), triglyceride (male: 131.57; female: 124.39) and fasting plasma glucose (male: 99.41; female: 94.06) are at higher level in the males than that of the females. But high-density lipoprotein cholesterol (male: 42.88; female: 48.42) is at higher level in the females than their counterpart. The males differ significantly with females in terms of age, BMI, waist-hip ratio, diastolic blood pressure, fasting plasma glucose and high-density lipoprotein cholesterol.

Means of traits are presented for the male in Table 14.2 separately for normal and individuals affected with Metabolic Syndrome (M.S.). The same have been shown in Figure 14.2. Systolic blood pressure

Table 14.2: Means of Traits in Normal and M.S. Males

Traits	*Male (n = 98)*						*t-value*
	Normal (n = 60)			*M.S. (n = 38)*			
	Mean	*S.D.*	*S.E.*	*Mean*	*S.D.*	*S.E.*	
Age (years)	44.85	12.26	1.58	50.84	16.91	2.74	1.89
BMI (kg/m^2)	22.80	3.71	0.48	23.50	3.16	0.51	1.00
WHR	0.93	0.07	0.01	0.93	0.08	0.01	0.34
SBP	119.30	0.08	0.01	137.97	27.69	4.49	4.16**
DBP	77.32	9.53	1.23	85.05	13.55	2.20	3.07**
TG (mg/dl)	125.90	40.80	5.27	140.54	40.84	6.62	1.73
FPG (mg/dl)	92.48	18.41	2.38	109.33	26.15	4.24	3.47**
HDL (mg/dl)	44.30	12.83	1.66	40.65	8.55	1.39	1.69

** Significant at 0.001 level of probability.

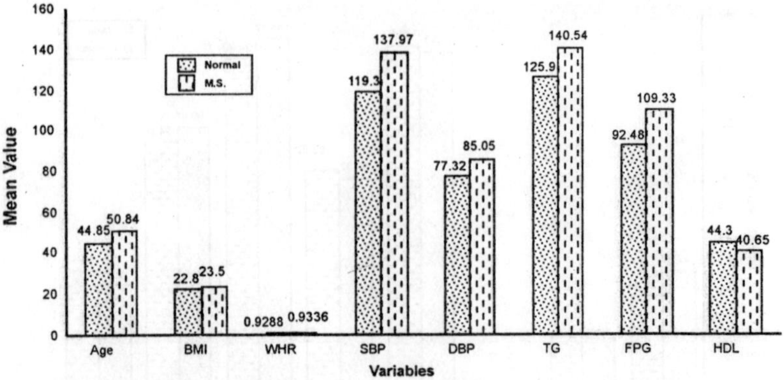

Fig. 14.2: Means of Variables in Normal and M.S. Males

(normal: 119.30; M.S.: 137.97), diastolic blood pressure (normal: 77.32; M.S.: 85.05) and fasting plasma glucose (normal: 92.48; M.S.: 109.33) are found to be considerably higher among the affected (i.e. M.S.) than that of the normal individuals. The individuals of these two sections (normal and M.S.) differ significantly with each other in respect of blood pressure (systolic and diastolic) and fasting plasma glucose. Side by side, among females the affected individuals (M.S.), however, show considerably higher mean value in case of almost all the traits than that of the normal individuals. BMI (normal: 22.76; M.S.: 28.52), waist-hip ratio (normal: 0.8594; M.S.: 0.9179), systolic blood pressure (normal: 126.17; M.S.: 138.12), diastolic blood pressure (normal: 81.49; M.S.: 92.06), triglyceride (normal: 122.59; M.S.: 130.09) and fasting plasma glucose (normal: 92.29; M.S.: 99.67) all are at higher level among the affected than that of the normal individuals. The individuals of these two sections are found to differ significantly with each other in respect of all these traits excepting triglyceride (Table 14.3 and Figure 14.3).

In Figure 14.4 the error bar charts are shown with 95 per cent C.I. for different traits (like BMI, waist-hip ratio, systolic blood pressure, diastolic blood pressure, fasting plasma glucose, triglyceride and high-density lipoprotein cholesterol) for both the groups and sexes. It is evident that there exist considerable differences between normal and M.S. individuals for both the sexes in terms of different traits. As these traits are quite self-explanatory it needs no further description.

The males and females subjects are presented in terms of experimental (affected individuals i.e. M.S.) and control group (normal

Table 14.3: Means of Traits in Normal and M.S. Females

Traits	*Female (n = 142)*						*t-value*
	Normal (n = 108)			*M.S. (n = 34)*			
	Mean	*S.D.*	*S.E.*	*Mean*	*S.D.*	*S.E.*	
Age (years)	38.18	11.66	1.12	39.26	12.73	2.18	0.44
BMI (kg/m^2)	22.76	3.44	0.33	28.52	2.79	0.48	9.93***
WHR	0.86	0.09	0.01	0.92	0.06	0.01	4.14***
SBP	126.17	19.29	1.86	138.12	24.52	4.20	2.60*
DBP	81.49	10.82	1.04	92.06	17.03	2.92	3.41***
TG (mg/dl)	122.59	43.08	4.14	130.09	42.54	7.29	0.89
FPG (mg/dl)	92.29	17.20	1.65	99.67	15.14	2.60	2.40**
HDL (mg/dl)	48.20	13.21	1.27	49.12	13.22	2.67	0.31

* Significant at 0.001 level of probability.
** Significant at 0.02 level of probability.
*** Significant at 0.01 level of probability.

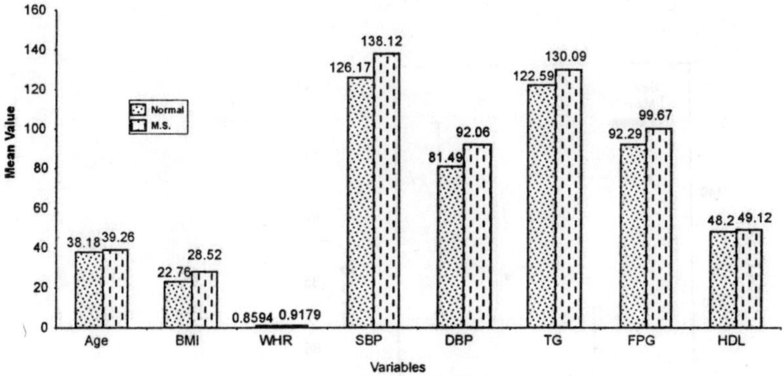

Fig. 14.3: Means of Variables in Normal and M.S. Females

individuals) in Tables 14.4 and 14.5 respectively. It is evident from both the Tables that the individuals of control group are certainly in better position in respect of almost all the traits related with metabolic syndrome. In males individuals with overweight (experimental: 31.58%; control: 25%), hypertension (experimental: 42.11%; control: 16.67%), high level of fasting sugar (experimental: 36.84%; control: 15%) and high level of triglyceride (experimental: 26.32%; control: 16.67%) are much lesser in frequency in control group than that of the experimental group (Table 14.4). Side by side, in the females individuals with overweight (experimental : 44.12%; control : 25.93%), central obesity (experimental : 52.94%; control : 32.41%), hypertension (experimental : 58.82%;

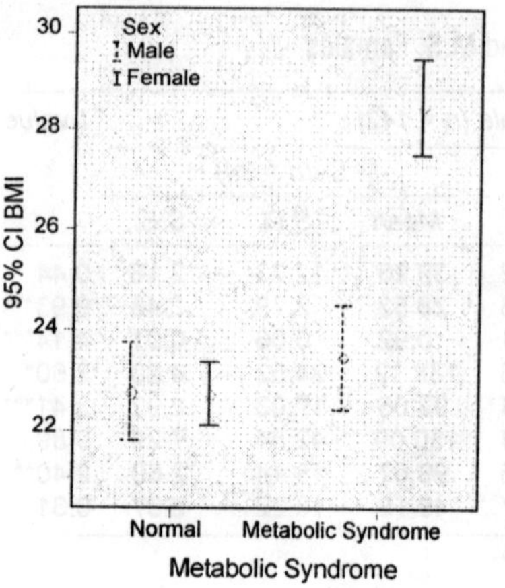
Sex
Male
Female
95% CI BMI
30
28
26
24
22
Normal
Metabolic Syndrome
Metabolic Syndrome

(a)

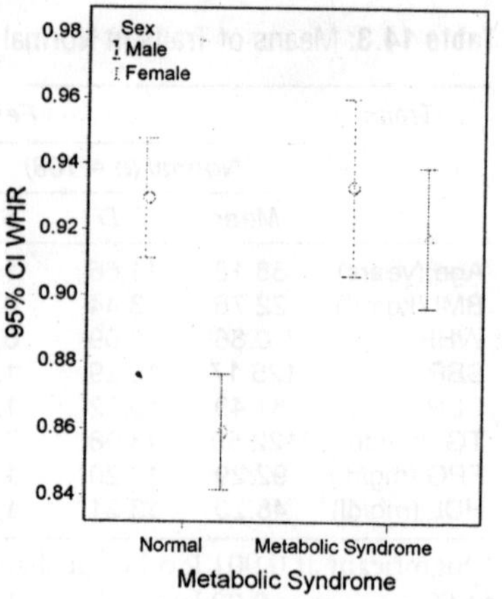
Sex
Male
Female
95% CI WHR
0.98
0.96
0.94
0.92
0.90
0.88
0.86
0.84
Normal
Metabolic Syndrome
Metabolic Syndrome

(b)

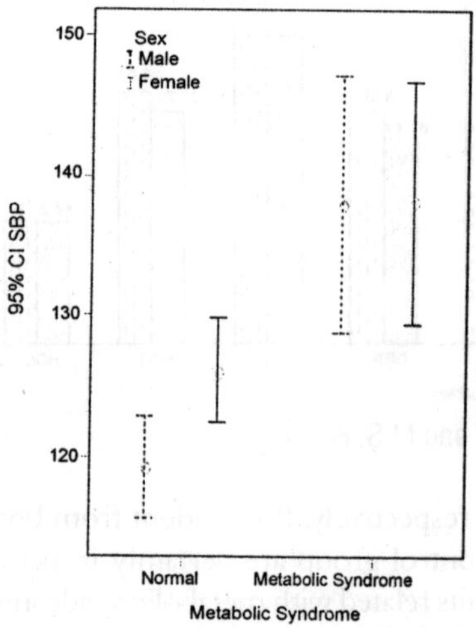
Sex
Male
Female
95% CI SBP
150
140
130
120
Normal
Metabolic Syndrome
Metabolic Syndrome

(c)

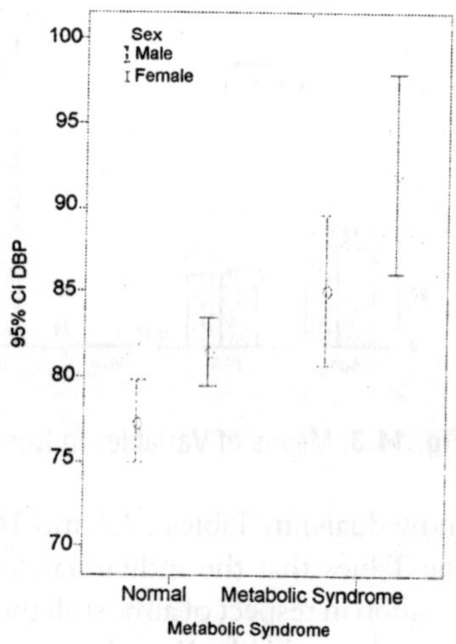
Sex
Male
Female
95% CI DBP
100
95
90
85
80
75
70
Normal
Metabolic Syndrome
Metabolic Syndrome

(d)

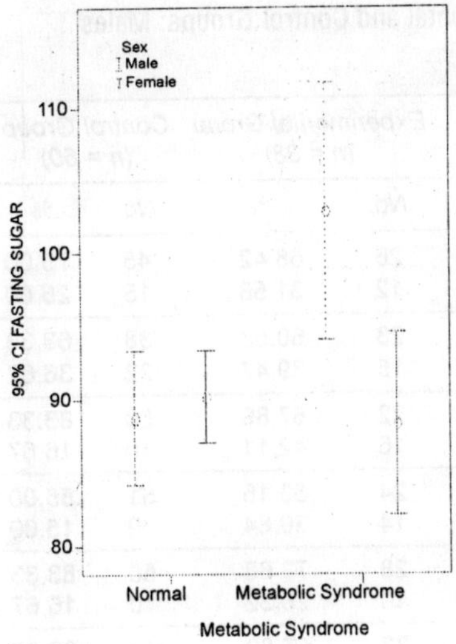

(e)

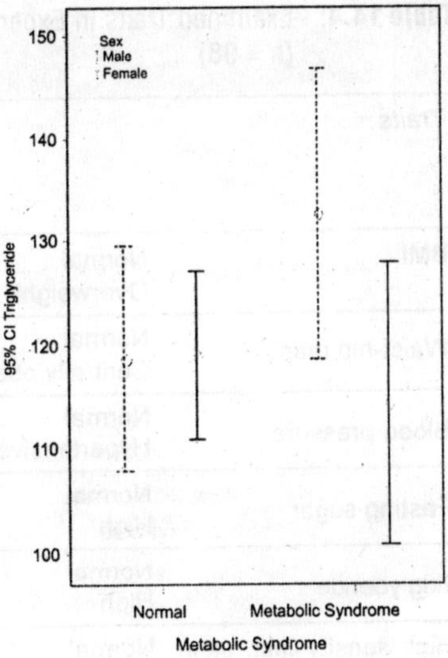

(f)

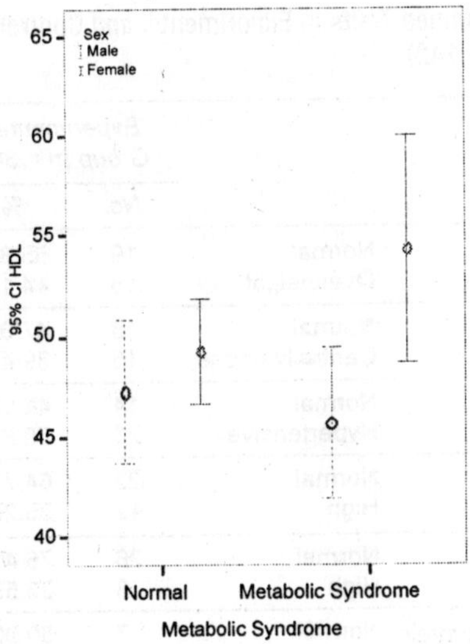

(g)

Fig. 14.4: Error Bar Chart Showing 95 per cent Confidence Interval of Mean value of BMI, WHR, SBP, DBP, TG, FPG and HDL

Table 14.4: Examined Traits in Experimental and Control Groups: Males (n = 98)

Traits		*Experimental Group (n = 38)*		*Control Group (n = 60)*	
		No.	*%*	*No.*	*%*
BMI	Normal	26	68.42	45	75.00
	Overweight	12	31.58	15	25.00
Waist-hip ratio	Normal	23	60.53	38	63.33
	Centrally obese	15	39.47	22	36.67
Blood pressure	Normal	22	67.89	50	83.33
	Hypertensive	16	42.11	10	16.67
Fasting sugar	Normal	24	63.16	51	85.00
	High	14	36.84	9	15.00
Triglyceride	Normal	28	73.68	50	83.33
	High	10	26.32	10	16.67
High density lipoprotein cholesterol	Normal	22	57.89	40	66.67
	High	16	42.51	20	33.33

Table 14.5: Examined Traits in Experimental and Control Groups: Females (n = 142)

Traits		*Experimental Group (n = 34)*		*Control Group (n = 108)*	
		No.	*%*	*No.*	*%*
BMI	Normal	19	55.88	80	74.07
	Overweight	15	44.12	28	25.93
Waist-hip ratio	Normal	16	47.06	73	67.59
	Centrally obese	15	39.47	22	36.67
Blood pressure	Normal	14	41.18	78	72.22
	Hypertensive	20	58.82	30	27.78
Fasting sugar	Normal	22	64.71	88	81.48
	High	12	35.29	20	18.52
Triglyceride	Normal	26	76.47	89	82.41
	High	8	23.53	19	17.59
High density lipoprotein cholesterol	Normal	17	50.00	76	70.37
	High	17	50.00	32	29.63

control : 27.78%), high level of fasting sugar (experimental : 35.29%; control : 18.52%) and high level of triglyceride (experimental : 23.53%; control : 17.59%) are much lesser in control group than that of the experimental group (Table 14.5).

The results of odds ratio and confidence interval of the risk of metabolic syndrome are presented in Tables 14.6 and 14.7 for males and females respectively. Factors like blood pressure and fasting sugar in males and BMI, WHR, blood pressure, fasting sugar and HDL showed significant relationship with this syndrome. It revealed for Table 14.6 that the males with hypertension were 0.2750 times more likely to have this syndrome (odds ratio = 0.2750; C.I. = 0.1079-0.7010). Side by side, males with high level of sugar were 0.3025 times more likely to have metabolic syndrome (odds ratio = 0.3025; C.I. = 0.1149-0.7963). Among the females in turn obese females were 0.4433 times more likely to have this syndrome (odds ratio = 0.4433; C.I. = 0.1987-0.9888). Females who are characterized with central obesity were 0.4262 times more likely to have this syndrome (odds ratio = 0.4262; C.I. = 0.1944-0.9344). Likely, females with hypertension (odds ratio = 0.2692;

Table 14.6: Results of Odds Ratios and Confidence Interval in Relation to Risk Factors: Males

Factors	*Reference Category*	*Odds Ratio*	*95% CI*	*Inference*
BMI Normal	High	0.7222	0.2937-1.7757	0.5045
WHR Normal	Centrally obese	0.8877	0.3848-2.0479	0.7080
Blood pressure Normal	Hypertensive	0.2750	0.1079-0.7010	7.7240*
Fasting sugar Normal	High	0.3025	0.1149-0.7963	6.1796*
Triglyceride Normal	High	0.5600	0.2078-1.5089	1.3335
HDL Normal	High	0.6875	0.2973-1.5898	0.7703

*Significant at 0.05 level of probability.

Table 14.7: Results of Odds Ratios and Confidence Interval in Relation to Risk Factors: Females

Factors	*Reference Category*	*Odds Ratio*	*95% CI*	*Inference*
BMI Normal	High	0.4433	0.1987-0.9888	4.0535*
WHR Normal	Centrally obese	0.4262	0.1944-0.9344	4.6608*
Blood pressure Normal	Hypertensive	0.2692	0.1207-0.6004	10.9254'
Fasting sugar Normal	High	0.4167	0.1773-0.9794	4.1687*
Triglyceride Normal	High	0.6938	0.2725-1.7661	0.5919
HDL Normal	High	0.4210	0.1913-0.9264	4.7480*

*Significant at 0.05 level of probability.

C.I. = 0.1207-0.6004), high plasma sugar (odds ratio = 0.4167; C.I. = 0.1773-0.9794) and high HDL (odds ratio = .4210; C.I. = 0.1913-0.9264) were more likely to have metabolic syndrome.

Prevalence of one or more of the metabolic abnormalities and co-occurrence of three of more of the components show overall 33 per cent with BMI and 29 per cent with WHR contribute as the measures of obesity (Table 14.8). Pair-wise correlations of the individual phenotypes indicate that components like: (i) BMI-WHR, (ii) BMI-DBP, (iii) WHR-DBP, (iv) SBP–DBP, and (v) SBP–HDL in males and components like: (i) WHR–FPG, (ii) SBP–DBP, and (iii) FPG–TG in females are significantly associated with each other, suggesting their co-morbidity in individuals. Thus obesity, hypertension and dyslipidemia in males and hypertension, dyslipidemia and plasma glucose in females appear to be major risk factors causing metabolic syndrome in Poundra Kshatriya population (Table 14.9).

Table 14.8: Prevalence of one or more Abnormalities

Traits	*No. of abnormalities in %±S.E.*				
	≥1	≥2	≥3	≥4	5
BMI as the measure of obesity	74.32±4.6	62.51±3.4	32.71±3.4	15.10±4.5	1.10±1.1
WHR as the measure of obesity	76.41±4.7	69.22±4.1	29.02±2.9	18.40±2.7	0.93±1.2

Male: Upper triangular matrix; Female: Lower triangular matrix.
*Significant at 0.05 level of probability.
** Significant at 0.01 level of probability.

Table 14.9: Values of Pearson Correlation Coefficients among Different Traits

Traits	*BMI*	*WHR*	*SBP*	*DBP*	*TG*	*FPG*	*HDL*
BMI	—	0.467**	0.141	0.322*	0.148	-0.192	-0.149
WHR	-0.089	—	0.315	0.342*	0.085	-0.025	0.111
SBP	0.042	0.111	—	0.839**	-0.082	-0.040	0.481**
DBP	0.199	-0.198	0.771**	—	-0.129	-0.115	0.479**
TG	-0.143	0.117	0.045	-0.002	—	0.066	-0.139
FPG	-0.008	-0.347*	-0.115	0.126	0.341*	—	0.092
HDL	0.189	0.064	0.031	0.072	0.008	0.233	—

Male: Upper triangular matrix; Female: Lower triangular matrix.
*Significant at 0.05 level of probability.
** Significant at 0.01 level of probability.

Discussion

Metabolic syndrome is a rising disease entity characterized by a combination of metabolic conditions. Obesity is one of the major underlying causes of the metabolic syndrome. The mechanisms whereby obesity elicits or worsens metabolic risk factors are not fully understood but several potential links exist. Obesity is accompanied by high plasma levels of non-esterified fatty acids that cause insulin resistance in skeletal muscle and overload the liver with lipid, producing fatty liver and atherogenic dyslipidemia (Grundy 2000). Comparative studies indicate that metabolic responses to obesity may be greater in South and East Asians that their Western counterparts at given body mass indices (Pan *ét al.* 2008). Naguyen *et al.* (2008) suggested an optimal BMI cut off of <25 kg/m^2 for 18 to 65 years old Chinese men and women. They found a slight increase in the BMI cut offs (~0.5 kg/m^2) among older compared with younger participants. Their findings were consistent with results from large-scale cross-sectional studies in Chinese and Indian populations (Bei, 2002, Wildman *et al.* 2004, Lin *et al.* 2002 and Mohan *et al.* 2007). In these studies, a BMI cut off-of 22-24 kg/m^2 was associated with increased prevalence of hypertension, diabetes mellitus, dyslipidemia, and cardiovascular diseases. Huxley *et al.* (2008), in a sample of 2,63,000 participants (73% Asians) from 21 cross-sectional studies in Australia and some Asian countries, also showed an optimal BMI cut-off of ~24 kg/m^2 for Asians.

Considering BMI cut-offs of <25 kg/m^2 in the present study we find mean BMI is 23.07 in male and 24.14 in female. Present findings thus corroborate the findings of others in Asian populations. Overall prevalence of metabolic syndrome is 30 per cent (39% in males and 24% in females) in this peri-urban population. This indicates a substantially high occurrence of metabolic syndrome among the males than the females. Thus, the males are more exposed to the risk factors of this disorder than their counterparts. Prevalence of one or more of the metabolic abnormalities and co-occurrence of three or more of the risk factors show overall 33 per cent with BMI and 29 per cent with WHR contribute as the measures of obesity. Risk factors most prevalent were obesity, hypertension and dyslipidemia in males and hypertension, dyslipidemia and plasma glucose in females.

Nutritional, demographic, epidemiological and socio-economic transitions are occurring in many developing countries. With improvement in economic situation in developing countries, increasing prevalence of obesity and the metabolic syndrome is seen in adults and particularly in children. The main causes are urbanization, nutrition transition, and reduced physical activity (Misra and Khurana 2008). It is generally believed that >> less oily-less fat–less consumption of junk food << considerably reduces the rate of all cause mortality and metabolic syndrome in any population. Therefore, it is intriguing that in spite of adherence to a relatively less stressful and high physical activity lifestyle pattern the prevalence of metabolic syndrome in this population is considerably high. It can be well assumed that due to the nearness to urban centre, Kolkata this population is undergoing changes in their lifestyle as well as dietary pattern.

The recent data show that one-fourth to one-third of urban population of India has the metabolic syndrome. Furthermore, the prevalence is 4.5-2 times higher in women compared with men. Interestingly, certain communities in India (e.g. Punjabi Bhatia community in North India) have inordinately high tendency to have obesity, T2DM, and the metabolic syndrome (cf. Misra and Khurana 2008). According to present study 39 per cent of the males and,24 per cent of the females are found to be affected by this syndrome. Findings of the present study are however, indicative of preponderance of males over females. Although the average value of waist circumference in South Asians is lower than other ethnic groups, abdominal adiposity is significantly more than white Caucasians (cf. Misra and Khurana 2008). Raji *et al.* (2001) showed that at similar value of BMI, migrant Asian Indians had significantly greater total abdominal fat and intra-abdominal fat with than white Caucasians in the United States. Findings of the present study show that 37.75 per cent males and 37.72 per cent females are centrally obese in this population. This indicates high per cent of central obesity among them.

Urbanization is the prime driver for nutrition transition and emergence of obesity, metabolic syndrome and other nutritionally controlled diseases in developing countries. The previously held view that people belonging to high SES are more predisposed to develop obesity in developing world is no longer tenable. The burden of obesity in developing countries shifts toward the people belonging to lower SES as the country's GDP increases, probably because scarcity of food and/or physically demanding lifestyle become less common, even in people belonging to low SES after the economy improves (Misra and Khurana 2008). India currently has one of the 10 fastest growth economies in the world. The Tenth Five Year Plan of India set a target of 8.0 per cent GDP growth for 2002-07 and 9.3 per cent in Eleventh Five Year Plan (2007-12). In accordance with this goal, the annual rate of growth of GDP has accelerated to 8 per cent in 2006-07, compared with 6.1 per cent per annum during 1990s. In context of the present study the impact of urbanization cannot be ruled out in this peri-urban population. These probably have played important role behind the high prevalence of metabolic syndrome among them. However, there is a need for comprehensive studies to assess changes in lifestyle and dietary patterns among the Poundra Kshatriya population.

Acknowledgement: This paper is based on the project entitled, "DNA Polymorphism and Diseases (Epidemiological Studies: Cardiac Diseases)", which was approved by the Anthropological Survey of India, Kolkata. Both the authors are grateful to the said Organization. The authors are also grateful to all the Poundra Kshatriya subjects who participated in this study.

References

Alberti, K.G. and P.Z. Zimmet 1998. For the WHO Consultation: Definition, Diagnosis and Classification of Diabetes Mellitus and its Complications. Part I: Diagnosis and Classification of Diabetes Mellitus, Provisional report of a WHO Consultation, *Diabet Med.* 15:539-53.

Bei, F.Z. 2002. Predictive Value of Body Mass Index and Waist Circumference for Risk factors of certain related Diseases in Chinese Adults: Study on Optimal cut-off points of Body Mass Index and Waist Circumference in China Adults, *Asia Pac J. Clin Nutr* 11 Suppl. 8:5685-93.

Deka, R. with N.S. Narancic, H. Xi, S. Turek, M. Cubrilo-Turek, D. Vrhovski-Hebrang, B. Janicijevic, A. Tomljenovic, L. Jin, R. Chakravorty and P. Rudan 2008. Metabolic Syndrome in an Island Population of the Eastern Adriatic Coast of Croatia, *Coll. Antropol* 32 (1) 85-91.

Gogia, A. and P.K. Agarwal 2006. Metabolic Syndrome, *Indian Journal of Medical Sciences* 60 (2) 72-81.

Grundy, S.M. 2000. Metabolic Complications of Obesity, *Endocrine* 13:155-165.

Haffner, S.M. with M.P. Stern, H.P. Hazuda, J.A. Pugh, J.K. Patterson and R.M. Malina 1986. Upper Body and Centralized Adiposity in Mexican Americans and non-Hispanic Whites: Relationship to Body Mass Index and other Behavioural and Demographic Variables, *Int J. Obes* 10:493-502.

Huxley, R. with W.P. James, F. Barzi, J.V. Patel, S.A. Lasker, P. Suriyawongpaisal, E. Janus, I. Caterson and P. Zimmet 2008. Ethnic Comparisons of the Cross-sectional Relationships between Measures of Body Size with Diabetes and Hypertension, *Obes Rev* 9:53-61.

Lin, W.Y. with L.T. Lee, C.Y. Chen, H. Lo, H.H. Hsia, I.L. Liu, R.S. Lin, W.Y. Shau and K.C. Huang 2002. Optimal cut-off Values for Obesity using Simple Anthropometric Indices to Predict Cardiovascular Risk Factors in Taiwan, *Int J. Obes Relet Metab Disord* 26:1232-8.

Misra, A. and L. Khurana 2008. Obesity and the Metabolic Syndrome in Developing Countries, *The Journal of Clinical Endocrinology and Metabolism* 93(1):9-30.

Misra A. with D. Chaudhary, N.K. Vikram, V. Mittal, J.R. Devi, R.M. Pandey, N. Khanna, R. Sharma and S. Peshin 2002. Insulin Resistance and Clustering of Atherogenic Risk factors in Women belonging to Low Socio-economic Strata in Urban Slums of North India, *Diabetes Res Clin Pract* 56:73-75.

Mohan, V. with M. Deepa, S. Farooq, K.M. Narayan, M. Datta and R. Deepa 2007. Anthropometric cut points for Identification of Cardiometabolic Risk factors in an Urban Asian Indian Population, *Metabolism* 56:961-8.

National Institute of Health 2001. *Third Report of the National Cholesterol Education Programme. Expart Panel on Detection, Evaluation and Treatment of High Blood Cholesterol in Adults (Adult Treatment Panel III),* National Institute of Health, NIH Publication 01-3670, Bethesda, MD, 2001.

Pan, W.H. with W.T. Yeh and L.C. Weng 2008. Epidemiology of Metabolic Syndrome in Asia. *Asia Pac J. Clin Nutr* 17, Suppl 1: 37-42.

Raji, A. with E.W. Seely, R.A. Arky and D.C. Simonson 2001. Body fat Distribution and Insulin resistance in Healthy Asian Indians and Caucasians, *J. Clin Endocrinol Metab* 86:5366-5371.

Reaven', G. 1988. Diabetes, 37:1595 (cf. Deka, R. with N.S. Narancic, H. Xi, S. Turek, M. Cubrilo-Turek, D. Vrhovski-Hebrang, B. Janicijevic, A. Tomljenovic, L. Jin, R. Chakravorty and P. Rudan 2008. Metabolic Syndrome in an Island Population of the Eastern Adriatic Coast of Croatia, *Coll. Antropol* 32 (1) 85-91.

Singh, K.S. 2008. *People of India. West Bengal, Vol. II.* Kolkata: Anthropological Survey of India.

Vega, G.L. 2001. Obesity, The Metabolic Syndrome and Cardiovascular Disease, *Am Heart J.* 142:1108-16.

Wasir J.S. and A. Misra 2004. The Metabolic Syndrome in Asian Indians: The Impact of Nutritional and Socio-economic Transition in India, *Metab Syndr Relat Disord* 2:14-23.

Wildman, R.P. with D. Gu, K. Reynolds, X. Duan and J. He 2004. Appropriate Body Mass Index and Waist Circumference cut-offs for Categorization of Overweight and Central Adiposity among Chinese Adults, *Am J. Clin Nutr* 80:1129-36.

15

Food Habits and Diseases: Some Observations

Shruti Agrawal and *Pratiti Ghosh*

Introduction

The 20th Annual World Diabetes Congress of the International Diabetic Federation revealed that India leads in the epidemic of diabetes. 50.8 million people here suffer from diabetes, followed by China (43.2 million) and the US (26.8 million). By 2010 almost 7 per cent of India's adult population will probably have the disease.

Though the present-day Bengalees and Biharees have evolved from a mixed culture, yet they are wound by some common factors. Their food is traditionally and ritualistically linked to carbohydrate-rich items, along with fat, which are commonly associated with Metabolic Syndrome (MS), Cardiovascular Disease (CVD) and type II diabetes mellitus (T2DM) (Hippisley-Cox 2009, Mackay 2009). Diabetes is an epidemic in India, with Kolkata scoring the third place, being the haven of @15 per cent diabetics (National Institute of Clinical Excellence 2004).

Objective: To extrapolate food habits to the etiology of the prevalent diseases.

Data Source: Survey of eating and lifestyle patterns of 700 Bengalee and 200 Biharee families were correlated with PubMed and hospital databases published in the last decade.

Results

Considering the culinary activities associated with rituals, festivals and mundane events-foods define an occasion. Birthdays are traditionally linked with *'payasam'* or modern day cakes; *Bijoya Dasami*, *Holi* and *Bhatriduj* or *Bhaidwitiya* are linked to *'mishti'*, *Pithe parbon* is linked to homemade sweetmeats. Visit to friends and relatives' house is as courteous with sweets as is the welcoming of the guest by the host. Socializing demands the size and amount of these to be more than the daily requirement. Religious activities, especially with Hinduism, are liberal with carbohydrates and detest protein-rich items to the extent of banning even lentils for the widows. Besides the fact that carbohydrates are comparatively cheap and easily available, rites-rituals and spirituality go hand in hand with the vegetarian and the non-baked items in the meal.

If the daily food consumption is assessed among the low income group of people, they take a variety of cereals ranging from rice, roti, suji, dalia, luchi, puffed rice and their preparations. They have Bengal gram, lentils, chhola dal, soya beans, chhola-matar, groundnut, poppy seeds, dates, mustard seeds and their preparations. They also consume different varieties of non-vegetarian protein and milk. Their variety of vegetable intake is rather poor, ranging from brinjal, to all parts of banana tree and those from the tuber group. Their access to fruit is limited to cucumber, banana and cheaper varieties of seasonal fruits. They consume more of sweets, biscuits, tea, especially, lemon tea.

Their total intake and frequency is low with scarce variation in daily pattern, leading to a lack of vitamins and minerals (WHO 2006). They have more of carbohydrates, less protein and moderate amounts of fat. They stuff the cooking with more of spices and condiments to induce a feeling of quick satisfaction. They have inadequate knowledge regarding the methods of cooking, hygiene and sanitation. They do not/cannot afford to give importance to fruits.

The middle income group of people, unlike their low income counterparts, consumes sufficient calories and enjoys variety of vegetables and fruits but it is the high income group who enjoy the most variety and their food has excess processed, polished foods, trans-fats and total calories. This is not true with the health conscious group, though.

Survey of diabetics according to income would show that the least affected ones are those earning Rs. 5000-10,000 p.m., but those earning less or more have a higher incidence of the disease. Considering Basal Metabolic Index (BMI) (Ryde'n 2007, Lisa *et al.*, 2008, Hippisley-Cox 2009) highest occurrence of CVD, MS and T2DM are observed in those with BMI in the range between 30-40, followed by those between 25-29.9 and surprisingly, low frequency is observed in those with BMI more than 40! It is known that obesity located in the central abdominal part of the body is statistically associated with a number of metabolic derangements including increasing insulin resistance in those genetically predisposed to NIDDM (Non-Insulin-Dependent Diabetes Mellitus).

Most of the diabetics are from the age group of 46-55 years of age; males have a higher propensity than females (Shai 2006, Rung 2009) those belonging to the business class are more affected than those in service or are doctors; and as expected, sedentary groups are eight-fold more affected than those with heavy activity level.

Regarding awareness of scientific knowledge among the masses, 55 per cent of the people know that it is the hormone insulin and not other hormones, which are related to diabetes (Sridhar 2000, Mullican 2009). 23 per cent know T2DM is related to inactivity and stress, 15 per cent think it is due to faulty food habits, whereas 45 per cent know it is due to all these factors. Regarding different ways to remain fit, 15 per cent believe avoiding fasts is beneficial, 29 per cent prefer to avoid feasting, 47 per cent think restricting fatty foods is a safe way and only 10 per cent know that erratic diet and lifestyle hampers health. Again, 32 per cent take restricted diet, 29 per cent take recourse to yoga and meditation, 15 per cent take a brisk walk and 25 per cent rely on medicines to remain fit. Most of the people (61%) take three meals a day, 22 per cent take four meals, 10 per cent take five meals and 5 per cent take two meals a day (Gray 2007, Link 2009).

Finally, the survey shows that 65 per cent of the diabetics could relate this disease to someone in the family, 48 per cent with family history of CVD but the rest could not correlate with the family tree. Most diabetics have blood pressure greater than normal and suffer from complications of coronary heart disease (Millett 2007). More men than women have waist to hip ratio greater than 1 and 0.8 respectively, i.e., metabolic syndrome.

Discussion

Worldwide data shows that about ten or more genes are implicated in the etiology of T2DM, CVD and MS (Kenealy 2008, Lee 2009). It has been observed that the Asians, rather the Indians or rather the Tamils and Bengalees have a high propensity of this disease. The final manifestation or the onset of the disease or its severity is influenced by dietary habits and lifestyle (sedentary and late night dining) which in turn are influenced by environment, tradition and peers (Nyamdorj 2009) Bengal harbours and germinates a huge population with these diseases (presently 15% of India's diabetics). Tracing back to their socio-economic conditions, food habits and general lifestyle, they incubate most conditions conducive to the undesirable form of expression of the related genes (Ni Mhurchu 2006, Burner 2009).

The ability of food to contribute to health management has long been recognized. Nutritional molecules have the ability to trigger interconnected molecular mechanisms in various tissues throughout the body. Yet, the prevalence of food related diseases such as obesity, T2DM and CHD are on the rise in specific parts of the world (Hitti 2006, Carter 2008, Savitz 2008).

It is being repeatedly seen, the drastically difference in responses between individuals to a given diet. Certain genes are dynamically but differentially transcribed in different tissues of the body in different ethnic populations (Yeo 2006, Lustman 2008). The human genome differs between persons by 1 per cent (Kousta 2006, Science Daily 2009). Certain non-lethal mutations are maintained in a population at 5 per cent level and are thus called polymorphisms. These single nucleotide polymorphisms (SNPs) contribute to minor individualistic difference that explains many aspects of nutrigenomics/pharmacogenomics, rather, the differential response to same drug or diet!

Although smoking, physical activity and toxins are capable of modulating health; it is our continuous exposure to foods throughout our lifetime that renders our diet the most important environmental factor challenging our biological system. Thus, unlike a drug which targets a specific dysfunctional gene or its product, to improve health, the nutritional industry manages health through a complex mixture of nutritional molecules (i.e. diet), each component with its own influence on the metabolism. So, in comparison to a medicinal compound, consuming a diet drastically increases the number of end-points that are capable of influencing phenotype, thus placing nutrition at a prime point. This would suggest tailored diet according to genetic make-up, rather, specific diet pattern in accordance with the most predominant polymorphism present in that ethnic community (*The Telegraph* 18th

May, 2005, ANI 2009). Adoption of a different diet pattern (combining the traditional with the foreign), may not always be beneficial, as the mundane habits and patterns of lifestyle differ between communities.

Conclusion

So, the present data suggests that none of the non-invasive parameters are absolutely or solely responsible for the diabetes syndrome. Worldwide genetic data proves that may be 10 different genes are implicated in the etiology of diabetes and it is precipitated by undesirable food habits and sedentary lifestyle. Some ethnic groups such as the Asians or rather the Indians are presently vying for the top position in the list of diabetics. The cause may be attributed to the excess simple carbohydrate intake due to inferior economic conditions; or socio-religious taboos; or excess protein and saturated fat intake due to affluent conditions leading to precipitous BMI. These combined with sedentary activity or stress or depression, are compounded with the existing modification in genomics or proteomics to result in alteration in metabolomics, which disrupts the homeostasis, manifesting as a disease in course of time.

References

Burner, T.W. and A.K. Rosenthal 2009. Diabetes and Rheumatic Diseases, *Current Opinion on Rheumatology,* 21(1): 50-4.

Link, Carol L. and John B. McKinlay. 2009. Disparities in the Prevalence of Diabetes: is it race/ethnicity or socio-economic status? Results from the Boston Area Community Health (BACH) Survey, *Ethnicity and Disease,* 19(1):13-18.

Carter, P.J. with W.S. Cutfield, P.L. Hofman, A.J. Gunn, D.A. Wilson, P.W. Reed and C. Jefferies 2008. Ethnicity and Social Deprivation Independently Influence Metabolic Control Children with Type-1 Diabetes, *Diabetologia*, 51(10):1835-42.

Millett, Christopher, Sonia Sexena, Anthea Ng, Arch Mainous *et al.* 2007. Socio-Economic Status, Ethnicity and Diabetes Management: Analysis of Time Trends Using the Health Survey for England, *Journal of Public Health*, 29(4):413-419.

Mullican, David R. with Carlos Lorenzo and Steven M. Haffner. 2009. Is Prehypertension a Risk Factor for the Development of type 2 Diabetes? *Diabetes Care,* 32(10):1870-1872.

Sridhar, G.R. 2000. Review on Human Genome Project and its impact on Diabetes Mellitus., *International Journal of Diabetes for Developed Countries*, 20(5):1822-1825.

Shai, Iris with Rui Jiang, Joann E. Manson, Meir J. Stampfer, Walter C. Willett, Graham A. Colditz and Frank B. Hu 2006. Ethnicity, Obesity and Risk of Type 2 Diabetes in Women-A 20-year follow-up study, *Diabetes Care*, 29: 1585-1590.

Gray, Jeremy with Christopher Millett, Sonia Sexena *et al.*, 2007. Ethnicity and Quality of Diabetes Care in a Health System with Universal Coverage: Population-Based Cross-sectional Survey in Primary Care, *Ethnicity and Quality of Diabetes Care* 28(10):1485-1489.

Rung, Johan with Stephane Cauchi *et al.* 2009. Genetic Variant near IRS1 is Associated with Type 2 Diabetes, Insulin Resistance and Hyperinsulinemia, *Nature Genetics,* 41:1110-1115.

Hippisley-Cox, Julia with Carol Coupland, John Robson and Peter Brindle 2009. Predicting Risk of Type 2 Diabetes in England and Wales: Prospective Derivation and Validation of QD Score, *BMJ* 338: b880.

Hippisley-Cox, Julia with Shaun O'Hanlon and Carol Coupland 2004. Association of Deprivation, Ethnicity and Sex with Quality Indicators for Diabetes: Population Based Survey of 53,000 Patients in Primary Care, *BMJ,* 329:1267-70.

Kenealy, T. with C.R. Elley, E. Robinson, D. Bramley, P.L. Drury, N.M. Kerse, S.A. Moyes Arroll 2008. An Association Between Ethnicity and Cardiovascular Outcomes for People with Type 2 Diabetes in New Zealand, *Diabetes Medline*, 25(11):1302-8.

Kousta, E. with Z. Efstathiadou, N.J. Lawrence, J.A. Jeffs and I.F. Godsland 2006. The Impact of Eethnicity on Glucose Regulation and the Metabolic Syndrome Following Gestational Diabetes, *Diabetologia*, 49(1):36-40.

Ryde'n, Lars *et al.*, and other members of The Task Force on Diabetes and Cardiovascular Diseases of the European Society of Cardiology (ESC) and of the European Association for the Study of Diabetes (EASD) 2007. Guidelines on Diabetes, Pre-Diabetes and Cardiovascular Diseases, *European Heart Journal*, 34(1):1378-83.

Lee, H.M. with S.J. Chung, V.A. Lopez, N.D. Wong 2009. Association of FVC and Total Mortality in US Adults with Metabolic Syndrome and Diabetes, Chest, 136(1): 171-6.

Lisa, K. with Richardson Mappsy, Leonard E. Egede and Martina Mueller 2008. Effect of Race/Ethnicity and Persistent Recognition of Depression on Mortality in Elderly Men with Type 2 Diabetes and Depression, *Diabetes Care*, 31:880-881.

Lustman, P.J. with S.M. Penckofer and R.E. Clouse 2008. Recent Advances in Understanding Depression in Adults with Diabetes, *Current Psychiatry Report*, 10(6):495-502.

Mackay, Meredith F. with Steven M. Haffner, Lynne E. Wagenknecht, Ralph B. Agostino and Anthony J.G. Hanley. 2009. Prediction of Type 2 Diabetes using Alternate Anthropometric Measures in a Multi-Ethnic Cohort–The insulin Resistance Atherosclerosis Study, *Diabetes Care*, 32: 956-958.

Hitti, Miranda 2006. Ethnicity Alters Diabetes Risks: Changes in Weight, Diet may affect Black, Asians and Hispanics Differently than Whites, *Webbed Health New,* 10 (6):786-89.

Ni Mhurchu, C. with V. Parag, M. Nakamura, A. Patel, A. Rodgers and T.H. Lam 2006. Body Mass Index and Risk of Diabetes Mellitus in the Asia-Pacific region: Asia Pacific Cohort Studies Collaboration, *Asia Pacific Journal of Clinical Nutrition*, 15(2):127-33.

Ni Mhurchu, C. with Q. Qiao, S. Soderberg, J.M. Pitkaniemi, P.Z. Zimmet, J.E. Shaw and K.G. Alberti 2009. BMI compared with Central Obesity Indicators as a Predictor of Diabetes Incidence in Mauritius, *Obesity-Silver Spring*, 17(2):342-8.

Savitz, D.A. with T.M. Janevic, S.M. Engel, J.S. Kaufman and A.H. Harring 2008. Ethnicity and Gestational Diabetes in New York City, 1995-2003, *BJOG*, 115(8):969-78.

Yeo, K.K. with B.C. Tai, D. Heng, J.M. Lee, S. Ma, K. Hughes, S.K. Chew and K.S. Chai 2006. Ethnicity Modifies the Association Between Diabetes Mellitus and Ischemic Heart Diseases in Chinese, Malays and Asian Indians living in Singapore, *Diabeologia*, 49(12); 2866-73.

16

Nutritional Status of a Primitive Tribe: The Bharias of Patalkot

Ratna Bhattacharya

1. Introduction

The author has extensively covered the remotest areas of Patalkot crater which is situated between 22°-24' and 22°-29' NL and between 78°-24' and 78°-50' EL. 79 sq. km. area inside this crater is very much steep, rugged, undulating and forest covered. The villages are at different depths of the crater and it is difficult to move from one village to the other through these ravines. The villages are communicated with each other only by narrow, tortuous and almost inaccessible footpaths. In Patalkot, the whole village has been (of the 12 villages) considered instead of using individual families for data analysis. About Nutrition, the diet of these people generally lack requirements of a well balanced diet, partly due to their ignorance and partly due to their poor economic conditions. As forest inhabitants, the Bharias of Patalkot depended on hunting and gathering for ages before Agriculture was thrust upon them. Even now, a part of their calories come from forests. Although, the forests appear lush, it does not have the density and abundance of edible resources to sustain human foragers over long periods.

The Bharias show a remarkable, even puzzling resilience on the impact of modernization, thereby kept their identity intact. Pressure from the Government has compelled them to live as a cultivator against their wish. Thus, their current way of life is in a state of Transition and Jeopardy.

PATAL (Kot), as the name implies, is in a true sense, a *Deep Crater* in Chhindwara district of M.P. A section of Bharia tribe have taken shelter in this crater out of fear and settled there because of forest and land resources. (Though inadequate in quantity)

With a view to assessing the Nutritional Status of the Bharias of Patalkot, the author intends to discuss only the concept of the "Land Carrying Capacity" of all the villages in Patalkot. Although, other techniques which are quite available and admissible, the author will not consider them in the present analysis.

2. Methodology

At the very outset, a rapport was made with the tribal community. The author did it with ease because of her stay with the Bharias within the Patalkot Crater. Preliminary Census Survey was conducted for collecting data on Population composition of the villages in Patalkot.

The study was based on a generalized model as recommended by the ICMR (Indian Council of Medical Research).

From daily average consumptions of different nutrients data were calculated using Food Composition Chart of the ICMR and FAO (Food and Agricultural Organization). Estimation of number of consumption units of a family is essentially based on calorie requirement of each of the members of the family determined by the age and sex as recommended by the FAO at an ambient temperature of 25°C. However, special emphasis was given on the reconstruction of Calorie Estimates for the adult members whose age ranges from 15 years to 45 years. (See Table 16.2)

Although, the estimation of calorie consumption based on recommendation of the FAO is slightly different than that of ICMR, the grand averaging technique has considerably minimized this difference.

For the accuracy of the study, Statistical Models and Inferences were drawn based on the collected data.

Although, Weight/Height index and Average Skinfold over Triceps is an important criterion for estimating the status of nutrition, the author has considered only FIVE different directions with a view to achieving the nutritional status of the Bharias of Patalkot.

3. Data Analysis

3.1 Land Carrying Capacity (LCC) of Patalkot and its Nutritional Status

LCC is the maximum size that an environment can support, i.e. the size at which resources, living space and so forth are sufficient enough to assure the maximum well-being of the numbers of the population. *In the present context it is the maximum number of persons that can be nourished from the available land resource.*

In the present context, LCC is the maximum number of individuals to be supported by its land resource. Here, "Supports" mean, the proper K.cal-need that has to be achieved by the individuals/village from the said land resource.

Mathematically, LCC = A/NK, where A = Available Land for Cultivation, N = Individual Land Requirement and K = Land Use Factor = A/U. Here, U = Land Utilized.

3.2 Status of Nutrition has been found from 5 (FIVE) Different Directions

1. If "N" > land consumed, Malnutrition results.
2. If "LCC" > population size, Nutrition results.
3. Kcal-requirement > Kcal-obtained from food, labour, service etc., the malnutrition results.
4. Income required to support the family/individual > Average Usable Income, Malnutrition results. But all the above 4 items are interrelated.
5. BASAL METABOLISM

3.3 Land Use Factor and Kcal Need per Person per Year

Land Use Factor is the Probability of Land Utilized for Cultivation.

While calculating the Kcal obtained from utilized land, it has been assumed that ***1400 Kcal*** has been obtained per acre from an infertile land of Patalkot area. Therefore, from 62.5 acre utilized land in Gudhichhatri village, total Kcal obtained = **62.5 × 1400 = 87500 Kcal per year** (*See* **Table 19.1** for Gudhichhatri Village).

Again, assuming **865 Kcal** as the average need per person per year in Indian context, for 173 persons in Gudhichhatri, the total need = **173 × 865 = 149645 Kcal/yr.** (*See* **Table 19.1**)

So, "N" (individual land required in *acre/person/year*) = (62.5 × 149645/173 × 87500) = 0.618 acre. This value has been kept constant for the whole Patalkot.

3.4 Individual Land Consumption

- Individual Land Consumption per year for Gudhichhatri village
  = 62.5 acre/173 = 0.361 acre/yr. (*See* column 8 of Table 19.1)
- Land Carrying Capacity (LCC) = A/NK = 166.61/0.618 × 2.67 = 100.97 ˜ 101 persons for Gudhichhatri Village.
  12 Bharia villages have been studied as shown in Table 16.1. From the FAO-Chart, age-wise Kcal-need and the calorific values of 100 grams of edible items, following data has been (Table 16.2) reconstructed in Patalkot area.
  Avg. Kcal Obtained/acre/yr Avg.Kcal obtd. from Land (in Kcal/person/yr.)
  =1530 Kcal/acre/year = 499.72 Kcal/person/year
  = 1400 Kcal/acre/year in an infertile land = 500 Kcal/person/year

4. Results and Discussion

- Table 16.1 shows that not a single village in Patalkot area is NUTRITIONED.
- Out of 12 villages, 5 are MALNUTRITIONED (M).
- 6 villages are SEVERELY MALNUTRITIONED (S.M.).
- The average Kcal obtained from Patalkot land = 500 Kcal/person/year which is just sufficient for BASAL METABOLISM but not adequate for proper Nutrition. In a developing country like India, at least 800 Kcal/person/yr. is needed for moderate nutrition.
- Because of unique environmental setting where the Bharias are living in isolation in a deep crater for hundreds of years, they are different in every aspect of adaptation and behavioural pattern from the other upland tribes. For this reason, the author tried to investigate certain specific phenomena which experienced a distinctively divergent ecological niche.

Table 16.1: Village-wise Population and LCC:

Village Name	*Popu-lation size*	*Land Available "A" acre*	*Land Utilized "U" acre*	*Land-use Factor K = A/U*	*Kcal Obtd/ Kcal Need*	*Indv land Reqd. in 'acre'/ person/ year "N"*	*Indv Land Consu-mption*	*LCC Remark = A/ NK*
Gudhi-S.M. Chhatri	173	166.61	62.5	2.67	87500/149645	0.618	0.361	101
Ghatlinga S.M.	167	240.64	90.0	2.673	126000/295830	"	0.263	146
Palani M	167	180.0	67.5	2.67	94500/144455	"	0.404	109
Gaildubba								
Ghana M	180	208.52	78.0	2.673	109200/155700	"	0.433	126
Saldhana-Kodia								
Dhurni S.M.	17	4.53	4.0	1.13	5600/14705	"	0.235	7
Malni-Domni								
Khamarpur-M	174	205.72	68.33	3.01	95662/150510	"	0.393	111
Sehra-Pachgol								
Jad Mandal						"		
Harrakachhar-M	145	247.47	72.04	3.44	100856/125425	"	0.497	116
Jhiran	7							
Chimtipur-M	66	43.76	25.53	1.71	35742/57090	"	0.387	41
Sukhabhand-	76	24.48	9.18	2.67	12852/65740	"	0.121	15
S.M.-Harramanu								
Ghogri Gujjai	13	5.23	3.15	1.66	4410/11245	"	0.242	5
S.M. Dongr								
Karem Rated	254	249.42	93.38	2.673	130725/219710	"	0.368	151
S.M								

M = Malnutritioned, S.M. = Severe Malnutritioned

Last column indicates the Nutritional Status of the persons of a village. In Gudhichhatri village, the available land would be able to feed 101 persons whereas its population size is 173. So, it can be inferred that the village as a whole is Severely Malnutritioned (S.M.) as marked in the last column.

Table 16.2: Reconstruction of "Kcal Chart" of FAO for PATALKOT Reconstructed from FAO

Items	*Calorific Value for 100g of edible portion*	*Age in Years*	*Calorie Requirement/day*	
			Male	*Female*
RICE	360	20-30 yrs.	3200	2300
Potato	80-100	30-40 yrs.	3104	2231
Cow–milk	68	40-50 yrs.	3008	2162
Pork	340-400	50-60 yrs.	2768	1990
Wheat	350	60-70 yrs.	2528	1817
Egg	590	70 & above	2208	1587
Vegetable Oil	884	1 year	1000 (Boy)	850 (Girl)
Molasses (*Cane*)	250	2 years	1600	1360
		4 years	1860	1581
		6 years	2160	1836
		8 years	2400	2040
		10 years	2640	2144
		12 years	2870	2200
		14 years	2950	2258
		15 years	3100	2290

- The Study of the Bharias was based on a model recommended by the Indian Council of Medical Research (ICMR). Daily Kcal-intake obtained from different nutrients, their Kcal-needs were calculated using food composition chart of the ICMR and Food and Agricultural Association (FAO). However, for accuracy, mathematics of statistics has been used for drawing the influences on Land Utilization, Carrying Capacity, Working Capacity, Nutritional and Economic Status.

5. Conclusion

All the Bharia villages are malnutritioned because of underutilization of Land for cultivation. Not a single village has LCC higher than its population size. In all the villages, land requirement for an individual ('N') is much higher than the land consumed by an individual.

All the villages of Patalkot have Carrying Capacity less than its corresponding Population size. Thereby indicating that the villages are either Malnutritioned (M) or Severely Malnutritioned (S.M.)

Only 3 Villages (Palani-Gaildubba, Ghana-Saldhana-Kodia and Jadmandal-Harrakachhar) are slightly better insofar as the Nutritional Status is concerned.

In these 3 villages the difference between the Individual Land Requirement (0.618) and Individual Land Consumption (0.404 for Palani Gaildubba, 0.433 for Ghana-Saldhana-Kodia and 0.497 for Jadmandal-Harrakachhar) is marginally less.

Therefore, as a whole, PATALKOT IS MALNUTRITIONED.

Although an integration of data on "Agricultural Produce", "Occupational Status" (i.e. labour, service etc.), "Nutrition" (i.e. Kcal) and the "Economic Condition" have been attempted out of which only the Nutritional Status of the Bharias of Patalkot has been taken as a focal theme of this present scheme of analysis.

Patalkot Villages are a marginal case insofar as 'Basal Metabolism' is concerned. The villagers of Patalkot consume 500 Kcal/person/year, just sufficient for the Basal–need.

Within the bounds of the present analysis the Bharias of Patalkot are in a very bad shape in the Nutritional Aspects.

6. Certain Remedies

- Excessive human intervention and absence of high-tech innovation is unable to produce that requisite yield to supplement the calorie deficiency.
- So, better tools, implements, advanced eco-friendly agricultural method have to be evolved to increase the yield and finally absence of human exploitation is a must.
- Sustained drive under a planned economy to supply "optimum diet" through "protective food" like dairy product, poultry, egg, meat etc.
- A social safety-net for these poorest of the poor segments of the society is to be incorporated. The World Bank has thus carried poverty assessment in all borrower countries.
- Intensive and extensive farming to increase production for this segment.
- Social forestry (Acacia, bamboo, cashew plantation can be introduced.

Acknowledgement: The author sincerely acknowledges the guidance of Dr. Ranjana Roy, Emeritus Professor, Deptt. of Anthropology, Calcutta University. This is a part of her Ph.D. Thesis.

References

Annual Action Plan, 1985-86, *Patalkot (Bharia) Development Agency*, Tamia, Dist. Chhindwara, M.P.

Bhattacharya, Ratna *et al.*, 2002. Resource Utilization Among the Bharias of Patalkot in Central India, *In* M.L. Patel (ed.) *Global Perception of Tribal Research in India*, New Delhi: Atlantic Publishers and Distributors.

Bose, N.K. 1971. *Tribal Life in India,* New Delhi, National Book Trust.

Dixit, D.N. 1983. *Plan for Development of Bharias of Patalkot (A Primitive Tribe),* Bhopal: Tribal Research and Development Inst.

Drysdale, T. 1881. *Census of India: Census of the Central Provinces,* Bombay: Educational Society's Press.

Gopalan, C. with Rama B.V. Shastri and S.C. Balsubramanium 1971. *Nutritive Value of Indian Foods,* Hyderabad: National, Inst. of Nutrition.

ICMR 1966. *The Nutritive Value of Indian Foods and the Planning of Satisfactory Diet*, Sp. Rep. Series. No. 42, pp. 8.

Keys, A. with J. Brozek, A. Henschel, O. Mickelsen and H.L. Taylor 1950. *The Biology of Human Starvation,* Minnesota: The University of Minnesota Press.

Roy, J.K. and B.C. Roy 1982. *Hunger and Physique, A Study of the Juang Population of Orissa,* Calcutta: Anthropological Survey of India.

Service, E.R. 1966. *The Hunters*, New Jersey: Prentice Hall Inc.

—— 1979. *The Hunters*, 2nd ed. Englewood Cliffs: N.J. Prentice Hall.

17

Reproductive Performance among the Namasudra: A Study on Location Distance

Haradhan Mondal

Introduction

India holds a special position in the world in terms of population. It is one of the oldest civilizations in the world. People have inhabited it thousands of years. No wonders, at present it constitutes one of the most crowded parts of the world. In order to check the growth of population it is essential to understand the process through which the fertility behaviour is regulated in different cultural groups. The norms, values, customs and taboos prevalent in a society regulate reproductive behaviour. To understand the fertility behaviour of any group, these norms and values must be pinpointed.

It is difficult to ascertain why people want more children as it is associated with economic, social and psychological considerations, which cannot be easily disentangled. The situation also varies from society to society and among individuals within a society. In many societies it is found that parent 'reproductive goals', where they exist, are based on the number of children expected to survive them and care for them in their old age, they must have in high mortality country (ESCAP 1988). Such a level of fertility is close to a biological ceiling for all practical purposes.

Reproductive patterns vary between two cultural groups, between communities of various socio-economic status even communities residing in different geographical settings. It is generally believed that availability of health care facilities diminishes with the geographic distances of the locations increases from the nearest urban centre. The Scheduled Castes, Scheduled Tribes and other backward castes from the economically weaker sections in the society. Numerically Namasudra are the second largest in West Bengal in the category of Scheduled Castes. Present study is an attempt to deal with various aspects of reproductive performance among the Namasudra population residing in three different locations of North 24-Parganas district of West Bengal.

Material and Methods

According to Bose (1975), besides agriculture navigating boats is also a traditional occupation of Namasudra. At present they are engaged in various occupations like cultivation, agricultural labour, day labour, bidi binding, hawkery, carpentry, driving, teaching, services in government and private enterprise, business of rice making, tailor, rickshaw/van puller etc.

Bongaon block of North 24-Parganas district is purposively selected which have predominated concentration of Namasudra population compared to other blocks of the district, to ensure maximum coverage of Namasudra community and to minimize the cost and time involved in the survey and to facilitate maximum utilization of the time available for research. The data of the present study were collected from three villages namely Purana Bongaon, Paschim Ramchandrapur and Kansona on the basis of their locations from the Sub-divisional Health Centre, situated in Bongaon town. These are as follows:

- Village I: Purana Bongaon—located nearer to the Sub-Divisional Health Centre (i.e. 3 km. far);
- Village II: Paschim Ramchandrapur—located far from the Sub-Divisional Health Centre (i.e. 7 km. far) and
- Village III: Kansona—located at a location furthest from the Health Centre (i.e. 12 km. far).

Information have been collected from 876 ever married women. Out of which 202 from Purana Bongaon, 426 from Paschim Ramchandrapur and 248 from Kansona have been identified for in-depth interview. Necessary information have been collected through structured schedules.

Results and Discussion

Altogether four twin births have been found among them. Out of these two cases of twins are recorded in Purana Bongaon. Side by side, in Kansona village also two cases are reported. But in Paschim Ramchandrapur there is no such case. Altogether there are three married women, who are found to be sterile. Out of these three married women one belongs to Purana Bongaon village and the rest other two belong to Kansona village.

In Table 17.1 number of mothers are shown according to villages. Altogether, 876 mothers are taken into consideration for the purpose of present study. Out of which 202 belong to Purana Bongaon and 426 belong to Paschim Ramchandrapur village, while the rest i.e. 248 mothers belong to village Kansona.

Table 17.1: Number of Mothers according to Villages

Village	*Total Number of Mothers*
Purana Bongaon	202
Paschim Ramchandrapur	426
Kansona	248
Total	**876**

It reveals that there is a u-turn in average live births with the increase in age at menarche among the studied population. Average live births are enumerated to be highest among the women who attained their menarche in 13-14 years age group and the lowest is recorded in 15 years and above age group. While, in 11-12 years age group an intermediate value is recorded in this context (Table 17.2). A more or less similar trend is noticed in case of three villages (Table 17.3). However, average number of deaths are found to be increasing with increase in age at menarche, which is true for the Namasudra residing in Kansona village. But in Purana Bongaon and Paschim Ramchandrapur village a dissimilar trend is noticed. In Purana Bongaon village lowest average of deaths is recorded in 13-14 years age group, while in Paschim Ramchandrapur the same is recorded in 15 years and above age group (Table 17.3).

Table 17.2: Reproductive Performance of Post-menopausal Women

Age at Menarchae (in years)	*No. of Mothers*	*Average no. of Pregnancies*	*Average no. of Deaths*	*Average Live Births*
11-12	57	6.32	0.13	6.01
13-14	111	6.34	0.14	6.12
15 and above	73	5.81	0.25	5.43
Total	**241**	**6.21**	**0.18**	**5.86**

Average number of live births of all the mothers are presented in Table 17.4 according to villages. It is interesting to note that average number of live births per mother increases in these villages as the geographical distance increases from the Block headquarters. Average number is recorded to be lowest in Purana Bongaon village (3.0841±0.1323) and highest in Kansona village (3.7137±0.1500), whereas in Paschim Ramchandrapur village (3.5446±0.1060) an intermediate value is recorded.

In Table 17.5 average live births of the Namasudra women is presented according to the age at marriage. It reveals that average of live births decreases with the increase in age at marriage, which is true for all the villages. However, the average live birth is found to be comparatively lower in Purana Bongaon village than other two villages. Side by side, these values are comparatively lower in Paschim Ramchandrapur than that of Kansona village.

Infant mortality for the Namasudra residing in three villages are presented in Table 17.6. It is interesting to note that like average live births in case of infant mortality also the percentage value increases in the villages as their geographical distance from the nearest urban centre increases. Infant mortality is found to be 5.07 per cent among the Namasudra. When the three villages are taken into consideration it is found to be lowest in Purana Bongaon (3.85%) and highest in Kansona village (6.30%), whereas in Paschim Ramchandrapur village an intermediate value (4.83%) is recorded. It is, however, important to note that in Kansona village the per cent of infant mortality is recorded to be much higher than Purana Bongaon and Paschim Ramchandrapur.

In Table 17.7 per cent of toddler (1-4 years) and under-5 mortality are presented. Per cent of toddler and under-5 mortality are 1.80 and 6.88 respectively among the Namasudra. Like infant mortality in case of toddler and under-5 mortality a similar trend is noticed. However,

Table 17.3: Reproductive Performance of Post-menopausal Women according to Villages

Age at menarche (in years)	*Purana Bongaon*			*Paschim Ramchandrapur*			*Kansona*		
	No. of mothers	*Average no. of deaths*	*Average live births*	*No. of mothers*	*Average no. of deaths*	*Average live births*	*No. of mothers*	*Average no. of deaths*	*Average live births*
11-12	9	0.14	5.89	27	0.12	6.01	19	0.14	6.02
13-14	23	0.12	6.17	54	0.32	6.34	34	0.28	6.72
15 and above	13	0.21	5.34	39	0.14	5.81	23	0.25	5.78
Total	**45**	**0.16**	**5.87**	**120**	**0.19**	**6.05**	**76**	**0.23**	**6.16**

Table 17.4: Average Live Births according to Villages

Village	*No. of Mothers*	*Total no. of Live Births*	*Average Live Births per Mother ± S.E.*
Purana Bongaon	202	623	3.0841±0.1323
Paschim Ramchandrapur	426	1510	3.5446±0.1060
Kansona	248	921	3.7137±0.1500
Total	**876**	**3054**	**3.4863±0.1231**

Table 17.5: Age at Marriage and Average Live Births among the Namasudra Women

Age of marriage (in years)	*Purana Bongaon*		*Paschim Ramchandrapur*		*Kansona*		*Total*	
	No. of mothers	*Average Live births*	*No. of mothers*	*Average live births*	*No. of mothers*	*Average live births*	*No. of mothers*	*Average live births*
upto 19	37	3.79	68	3.95	49	4.10	176	3.89
20-24	158	3.11	347	3.31	196	3.95	668	3.33
25 and above	7	2.41	11	2.37	3	2.78	32	2.31
Total	**202**	**3.10**	**426**	**3.21**	**248**	**3.61**	**876**	**3.17**

Table 17.6: Infant Mortality according to Villages

Village	*No. of mothers*	*Total no. of live births*	*Neonatal deaths*	*Post neonatal deaths*	*Total infant deaths*	*Infant mortality (in %)*
Purana Bongaon	202	623	5 (0.80)	19 (3.05)	24	3.85
Paschim Ramchandrapur	426	1510	43 (2.85)	30 (1.99)	73	4.83
Kansona	248	921	26 (2.82)	32 (3.47)	58	6.30
Total	**876**	**3054**	**74 (2.42)**	**81 (2.65)**	**155**	**5.07**

Note: Figures in parenthesis indicate percentage values.

in Kansona village both the toddler and under-5 mortality are found to be much higher than other two villages.

Table 17.7: Child Mortality according to Villages

Village	*No. of mothers*	*Total no. of live births*	*Toddler mortality (1-4 years)*	*Toddler mortality (in %)*	*Under-5 mortality*	*Under-5 mortality (in %)*
Purana Bongaon	202	623	7	1.12	31	4.97
Paschim Ramchandrapur	426	1510	19	1.26	92	6.09
Kansona	248	921	29	3.15	87	9.45
Total	**876**	**3054**	**55**	**1.80**	**210**	**6.88**

Pregnancy wastage among the Namasudra is shown in Table 17.8 for three villages. This percentage value is recorded to be highest in Paschim Ramchandrapur (2.17) and lowest in Purana Bongaon village (1.58). In village Kansona, however, slightly lower per cent (2.54) of pregnancy wastage is recorded than that of village Paschim Ramchandrapur. When the mean number of conception is taken into consideration lowest average is recorded in village Purana Bongaon (3.13) and highest is in village Kansona (3.81), whereas village Paschim Ramchandrapur stands in between (3.64) in this respect.

Table 17.8: Pregnancy Wastage according to Villages

Village	*No. of mothers*	*No. of conception*	*Mean conception*	*No. of abortion*	*No. of still birth*	*Total pregnancy wastage*	*Pregnancy wastage (in %)*
Purana Bongaon	202	633	3.13	3 (0.47)	7 (1.11)	10	1.58
Paschim Ramchandrapur	426	1552	3.64	29 (1.87)	13 (0.84)	42	2.71
Kansona	248	945	3.81	11 (1.16)	13 (1.38)	24	2.54
Total	**876**	**3130**	**3.57**	**43 (1.37)**	**33 (1.05)**	**76**	**2.43**

Note: Figures in parenthesis indicate percentage values.

When the binomial test of equality of proportions is performed for infant, toddler and under-5 mortality in three villages it is found that there is significant difference between villages .Purana Bongaon and Kansona is case of these three mortalities. Side by side between Paschim

Ramchandrapur and Kansona significant difference is noticed in case of toddler and under-5 mortality. But between Purana Bongaon and Paschim Ramchandrapur there is no significant difference in case of all three mortalities (Table 17.9).

Observation

Rele (1982) says that the survival and growth of any family or a closed social group depends intrinsically upon the level of fertility in relation to mortality. When the rate of infant mortality is calculated it is found that this rate is 50.75 per 1000 live births among the Namasudra which is comparatively lower than West Bengal State level data (i.e. 53 per 1000 live births). But the same is much lower than the Raj Gond (Tiwari *et al.* 2002) and Ladiya (Adak 2001) of Madhya Pradesh, Khampti of Arunachal Pradesh (Chowdhury *et al.* 1994) and Hajong of Meghalaya (Adak *et al.* 1999).

Mean of live birth among the Namasudra is found to be 3.49, which ranges from 3.08 to 3.71 in three locations. It reveals that the level of fertility increases among the Namasudra as the geographic distance of their location increases from the sub-divisional health centre. This is true in case of mortality rates also. When the rate of infant mortality among the Namasudra is compared with the national level data it is found that this rate is considerably lower among them than that our national average. This is true for the Namasudra residing in three different locations. However, when the infant mortality rate of the study population is compared with the state level data it is noticed that this is considerably lower among the Namasudra residing in Purana Bongaon and Paschim Ramchandrapur but considerably higher in Kansona village than that of the West Bengal State level data.

Antenatal care can contribute significantly to the reduction of morbidity as well as moratalities because besides offspring medical care it includes advice on the correct diet and provision of necessary medicine to pregnant women (Nair *et al.* 2000). Infant mortality rate is always used as a reliable and sensitive indicator of health status in a community. Low rate of infant mortality among the Namasudra of Purana Bongaon reflects a better standard of health as well as better acceptance of antenatal care by them. Side by side, its high rate in Kansona reflects a poor standard of health among the study population. However, Namasudra of Paschim Ramchandrapur stands in between in this respect.

Table 17.9: Binomial Test of Equality of Proportion on Infant, Toddler and under-5 Mortality

Village	*Infant mortality*			*Toddler mortality*			*Under-5 mortality*		
	T_1	T_2	*Inference*	T_1	T_2	*Inference*	T_1	T_2	*Inference*
Purana Bongaon *vs* Paschim Ramchandrapur	0.0098	0.0100	N.S.	0.0014	0.0052	N.S.	0.0112	0.0111	N.S.
Purana Bongaon *vs* Kansona	0.0245	0.0116	S.	0.0203	0.0078	S.	0.0447	0.0138	S.
Paschim Ramchandrapur *vs* Kansona	0.0147	0.0096	N.S.	0.0189	0.0059	S.	0.0336	0.0111	S.

N.S.: Non-Significant; S: Significant

References

Adak, D.K. 2001. A study of the Phenomenon of Demographic Transition among the Ladiya of Madhya Pradesh, *Antrhopologie* XXX/2-2:241-242.

Adak, D.K. with S. Sen Choudhury and S. Choudhury 1999. The Hajong of Meghalaya: A study on some Demographic aspects, *Arunachal University Research Journal* 2:35-45.

Bose, N.K. 1975. *The Structure of Hindu Society*, New Delhi: Orient Longman Ltd.

Chowdhury, D. with M.C. Behera and D.K. Adak. 1994. Some Bio-demographic aspects of the Khampti and its Demographic Transition, *In* S. Mukherjee, F.I. Hussain, P. Chakraborty and G. Das (eds.), *Demographic Profile of North East India*. New Delhi: Omsons Publications.

ESCAP 1988. Infant and Child Mortality: The Implications for Fertility Behaviour, *Population Research Leads*, No. 29, ESCAP, Bangkok.

Nair, P.M. with S.A. Chandran and A. Shaw 2000. The effect of Maternal Health Programmes on Infant and Child Survival in India, *J. Fam Welf* 46:61-63.

Rele, J.R. 1982. Trends and Differentials in Fertility, *In* Population of India, Country Monograph Series. No. 10. United Nations, New York.

Tiwari, M.K. with R. Chakraborty, A. Gupta and D.K. Adak 2002. The Raj Gond of Sagar District, M.P.: A Demographic Study, *In* D.K. Adak, B. Bhattacharya, R. Ghosh (eds.) *Demography and Health Profile of the Tribals (A Study of M. P.)*, Delhi: Anmol Publications.

18

Etiological Factors, Assisted Reproduction and Pregnancy Outcome: A Retrospective Observation Among Infertile Couples

Amlan K. Ray, Samiran Bisai, Kaushik Bose, Shraboni Ray, M. Roychoudhury and *J. Bhattacharya*

Introduction

Infertility is recognized worldwide as a public health issue by the World Health Organization (WHO) (Vayena *et al.* 2001). Its prevalence within the 12-month period ranges from 3.5 per cent to 16.7 per cent in developed countries and from 6.9 per cent to 9.3 per cent in developing countries with an average prevalence of 9 per cent (Boivin *et al.*, 2007), particularly 5 per cent in Andhra Pradesh, India (Unisa 1999) 15.1 per cent in Indian Kashmir (Zarger *et al.*, 1997). Tubal occlusion, Polycystic Ovaries (PCO), endometriosis, Poor Ovarian Reserve (POR), unexplained infertility and male factors are attributable to the infertility affecting both male and female which eventually causes 'childlessness' (no child after a given period of marriage) (Stephen and Chandra 1998, Larsen 2005). Application of Assisted Reproductive Technologies (ART) on such couples could be the reasonable option for achieving the pregnancy.

The ART is a procedure, which handles the human oocytes and sperm or embryos in In-Vitro condition for establishing a pregnancy

(Hochschild 2006). The application of such technology is an effective device in increasing rate of pregnancy for an infertile couple worldwide. The World Health Organization (WHO) terms infertility as the incapability to achieve pregnancy in spite of unprotected intercourse for a period of more than 12 months (WHO Manual 2000, Evers 2002, Zegers-Hochschild *et al.*, 2006, Schmidt 2006). There are more than 70 million couples suffering from infertility worldwide (Ombelet *et al.*, 2008, Inhorn 2003). Several biological and endocrinological factors are attributed to infertility, among them, the tubal occlusion which is by far the most common cause of infertility affects around 25 per cent (Jones 2005), Endometriosis (development of the endometrium tissue in outside the utero) affects 0.5-5 per cent (Ozkans Mur *et al.*, 2008), PCO—a heterogeneous endocrine/metabolic disorder, whose main features contain androgen excess, ovulatory dysfunction, and polycystic ovaries (Azziz 2007), which affects 5-10 per cent of women in their reproductive age (Diamanti-Kandarakis and Dunaif 1996, Gleicher and Barad 2006, Hart 2008, Cocksedge 2008). Male factor is on rise to the tune of 40 per cent and almost becomes a spermatogenic failure. (Visser and Repping 2010). According to the WHO, that the normal sperm concentration should be of >20 × 106/ml with >50 per cent of progressively motile sperm and presence of sperm with standard (no parameters provided) morphology (World Health Organization 1999). The failure to achieve this level is termed as male infertility.

One more factor is Poor Ovarian Reserve (POR), which means the remaining primordial, and resting follicles (Gougeon, 1996) into the ovary (Broekmans *et al.*, 2006) causes infertility. Etiology of POR may be due to early menopause, infection at the reproductive organ and other metabolic disorders and older age. The presence of antral follicles in the ovary is less than 5 (Klinkert *et al.*, 2004; Klinkert *et al.*, 2005) are the signs of this condition.

Women in their reproductive age are likely to be affected with genital tuberculosis when it infects the genital tract. This is called genital TB (Macaluso 2010) is stated to be a major factor for female infertility (Parikh *et al.*, 1997). In the woman, it causes tuberculous endomteritis (infection of the uterus) and salpingitis (infection of the fallopian tubes). This infection can often be silent, may not cause any symptom. Diagnosis will only be possible through PCR (Polymerase Chain Reaction) test which can pick up minute quantities of DNA from the 2nd day of period is unique to the tubercle bacillus.

Cryopreservation technique is a part of ART procedure where freezing and storage of gametes and embryos (Hochschild 2006) under-196°C in liquid Nitrogen takes place. The embryo thawed from this technique is Cryopreserved Embryo (CPE). Through this technique, an infertile couple can have subsequent try of CPE transfer to get the chances of pregnancy.

The current study was undertaken to find out the pregnancy outcome from the factors causing infertility with the application of ART in a sample of the population of an IVF clinic to investigate the association of both IVF (In-Vitro Fertilization) ET (Embryo Transfer) and CPE (Cryopreserved Embryo) transfer. The study further analyses the pregnancy of couples with different age categories and affected with genital tuberculosis.

Materials and Method

Study Population

Couples were predominantly Hindu of different districts of West Bengal belonging to middle income group. This group of couples either comes through referrals from gynecologists, patient-to-patient reference or through newspapers. The couples were selected after having carefully counselled before starting the IVF treatment.

Study Area and Data Collections

A retrospective study was conducted in Jodhpur Park IVF Clinic in Kolkata City, the provincial capital of West Bengal. This study was carried out retrospectively between January-December, 2008. A total number of 138 females within the age group of 20 to 49 years comprising 136 cycles were taken in 3 different sub-divisions. Data were collected from the registry of IVF procedure after documenting the report of β-hCG (Human Chorionic Gonadotropin) (marker of clinical pregnancy) in February 2009.

Statistical Analyses

All statistical analyses were undertaken using the Statistical Package for Social Sciences (SPSS). Significance level was set at $p < 0.05$.

Results

The distribution of the etiological factors is presented in Table 18.1. Of the 138 females evaluated, 7 factors were identified. Among them, tubal factors accounted for 23.91 per cent as the most common cause of the infertility. Other factors included unexplained which accounted for 10.14 per cent. Male factors accounted for 22.46 per cent, almost similar to tubal factors. It is important to note that male and female factors together accounted for 12.31 per cent. Metabolic disorders like endometriosis (11.59%), PCO (6.52%), Poor Ovarian Reserve (5.07%) and others (7.97%) are directly or indirectly associated with infertility (Figure 18.1).

Table 18.1: The Distribution of the Etiological Factors of the Studied Subjects

Etiological Factors	*n (%)*
Unexplained	14 (10.14)
Tubal	33 (23.91)
Male	31 (22.46)
Male + Female	17 (12.31)
PCOs	9 (6.52)
Endometriosis	16 (11.59)
POR	7 (5.07)
Others	11 (7.97)
Total	**138 (100)**

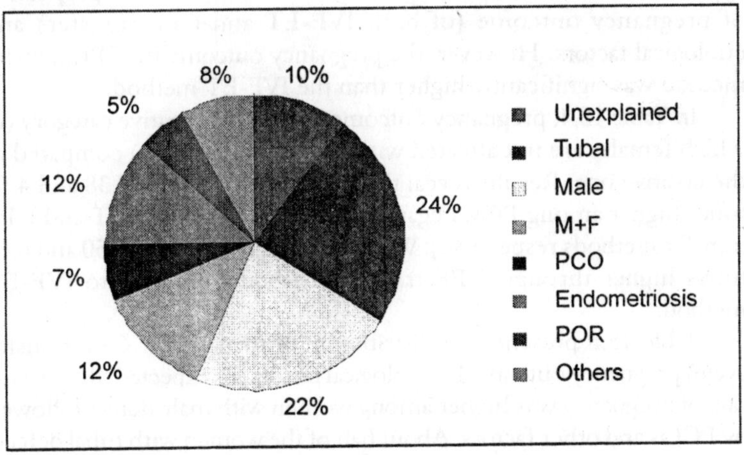

Fig. 18.1: The Chart showing the Distribution of Etiological Factors

The age group distribution over pregnancy outcome is presented in Table 18.2. Although the proportion of pregnancy outcome is featured in 30-34 years age group but age variation of pregnancy outcome found no significant differences. Moreover, the pregnancy outcome by CPE method in age group of 30-34 years and age combined was significantly higher than IVF-ET method.

Table 18.2: Age Group Distribution of Pregnancy Outcome by Assisted Reproductive Technology

Female Age	*Total Female Studied*	*IVF-ET*	*Pregnancy Outcome*	*CPE*	*Pregnancy Outcome*
20-29	36* (33)	21	8 (38.1)	12	7 (58.3)
30-34	65** (63)	46	18 (39.1)^	17	13 (76.5)^
35-49	37** (35)	20	7 (35.0)	15	8 (53.3)
Total	**138 (131)**	**87**	**33 (37.9)^^**	**44**	**28 (63.6)^^**

Note: IVF-ET = In-Vitro Fertilization, CPE = Cryopreserved embryo transfer.

★ 3 Subject excluded, ★★2 Subject excluded.

^ Significant difference: **chi-square (x^2) = 6.92, df = 1, p = 0.0053.**

^ ^ Significant difference: **chi-square (x^2) = 7.76, df = 1, p = 0.0053.**

In Table 18.3, 7 factors are clubbed together under 4 categories; pregnancy outcome against CPE is better than only IVF-ET with the application of ART. There was no significant difference in proportion of pregnancy outcome (of both IVF-ET and CPE transfer) and etiological factors. However, the pregnancy outcome by CPE transfer method was significantly higher than the IVF-ET method.

In Table 18.4, pregnancy outcome is better in negative category (in which females are not affected with genital tuberculosis) compared to the positive one. Results reveal that the success rate was 2.38 and 4.50 times higher among PCR negative women through IVF-ET and CPE transfer methods respectively. While, the success rate was 3.50 and 6.61 times higher through CPE transfer method compared to IVF-ET method.

Table 18.5 presents the distribution of total (1st + CPE transfer cycle) pregnancy outcome by etiological factors. As expected, the success rate of pregnancy was higher among women with male defect followed by PCOs and other factors. About half of the women with tubal defects have achieved clinical pregnancy. However, the proportion of pregnancy outcome was similar among couples suffered by POR and unexplained factors. In contrast, low success rate was noted among women suffered by endometriosis (Figure 18.2).

Table 18.3: Distribution of Pregnancy Outcome Related to Etiological Factors

Etiological Factors	*IVF-ET*	*Pregnancy Outcome*	*CPE transfer*	*Pregnancy Outcome*
Unexplained	8	4 (50.0)	4	2 (50.0)
Female	46	14 (30.4)	26	19 (73.0)*
Male	22	12 (54.5)	8	5 (62.5)
Male + Female	11	4 (36.4)	8	3 (37.5)
Total	**87**	**34 (39.1)**	**46**	**29 (63.0)****

Note: IVF-ET = In-Vitro Fertilization, CPE = Cryopreserved embryo transfer.

Figure in the parenthesis is percentage.

*Significant difference: **chi-square (x^2) = 12.17, df p = 0.0006.**

Significant difference: **chi-square (x^2) = 6.93, df = 1, p = 0.0084.

Table 18.4: Pregnancy Outcome through Assisted Reproductive Technology of PCR Positive and PCR Negative Women

PCR	*IVF-ET*	*Pregnancy Outcome*	*CPE Transfer*	*Pregnancy Outcome*	*Odds Ratio (95% CI)*
Positive*	9	2 (22.2)	24	12 (50.0)	3.50 (0.60-20.41)
Negative	79	32 (40.5)	22	18 (81.8)	6.61 (2.05-21.36)
Odds Ratio (CI)	2.38 (0.46-12.22)		4.50 (1.17-17.30)		

PCR = Polymerase Chain Reaction. *Reference category.

Table 18.5: Etiological Distribution of Pregnancy Outcome in Total (Fresh Cycle + CPE Transfer Cycle)

Diagnostic category	*Number of couples*	*Proportion of couples (%)*	*Pregnancy outcome in total (1st + CPE transfer Cycle)*
Unexplained	14	10.14	6 (42.86)
Tubal Factor	33	23.91	16 (48.48)
Male defect	31	22.46	20 (64.52)
PCOs	9	6.52	5 (55.55)
Endometriosis	16	11.59	3 (18.75)
POR	7	5.07	3 (42.86)
Male + Female	17	12.31	7 (41.18)
Others	11	7.97	6 (54.55)
Total	**138**	**100**	**66 (47.83)**

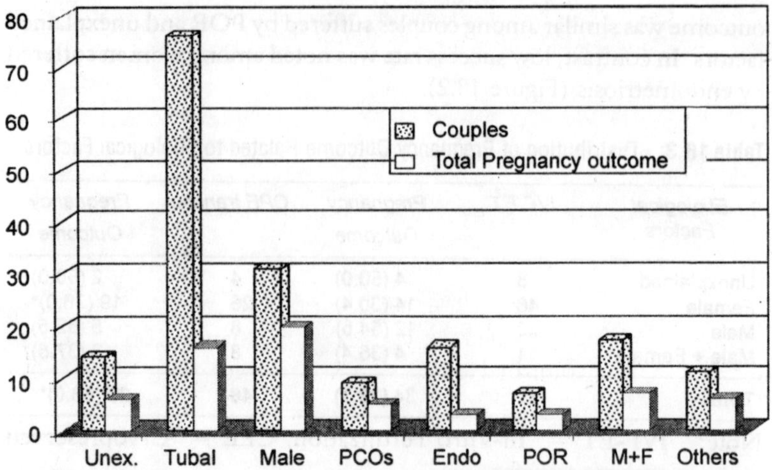

Figure 18.2: Total (Fresh Cycle + CPE Transfer Cycle) Pregnancy Outcome of Etiological Factors.

Discussion

Females of 30-34 years of age (comprise about 47% of 138 females) achieved 48 per cent pregnancy through ART compared to other two categories, as indicated in the Table 18.2 irrespective of the duration of infertility. It seems that the age of female is an important factor when IVF is likely to be suggested (Dicker *et al.*, 1991). Apart from its relation to age, female factor is also related to lifestyle, environmental factors and pathological events (Spira 1986).

Indian women suffer from infertility due to genital tuberculosis without any signs and symptoms (Dam 2006). After screening of clinic population, genital tuberculosis affected females are undergone anti-bacterial treatment before IVF protocol. Since this could also cause the infection in the fallopian tube (Singh *et al.*, 2008) and other part of the reproductive organ hence this is kept outside the purview of the etiological factors. Tubal damage is likely to have a poor prognosis for natural conception and is also caused due to endometriosis, PCO. In that case, IVF-ET is the preferred option (Hull 1985).

One of the interesting features in both male and female infertility is unexplained. The longer the duration of the treatment is likely to increase the lesser chances of pregnancy outcome. The better option is IVF-ET, if it fails, than CPE transfer is the subsequent option.

In the overall distribution of the sample, the proportion of tubal factors is comparable with the world data followed by the male factor.

However, our study is limited by virtue of small sample size. The results of the present study demonstrated some differences, though they were not significant. A much larger sample size could highlight significant differences. However, the data presented here can be utilized for comparisons with other existing clinical data.

Conclusion

The present study revealed that the overall pregnancy is on higher side in CPE transfer compared to IVF-ET in the mid-age group. PCR treated couples after the treatment offer lower pregnancy rate compared to the non-PCR. Whether the application of ART would be a solution to infertility could be proved in large-scale study in the population. Future studies could explore more entrants of types of factors attributed to infertility.

Women with poor ovarian reserve may have chances of conception with donated oocytes which is higher in comparison with the young women conceiving naturally. Assisted reproductive technologies are considered to be 'the ultimate salvation for these couples' (Baor 2005) when all attempts for achieving natural conception are failed. Given the fundamental importance of childless couple, suffered by various etiological factors, the application of ART to offer full term pregnancy instead of treating the disease may have an implication for childlessness.

Acknowledgements: The authors thank the staff of IIRC, Kolkata and scholars of the Department of Anthropology, Vidyasagar University for their technical assistance. We also thank Dr. Tuhin K. Das and Dr. D. Lohar of Jadavpur University for their selected comments.

References

Azziz, Ricardo (ed.).2007. *The Polycystic Ovary Syndrome: Current Concepts on Pathogenesis and Clinical Care,* New Delhi: Springer (India) Private Limited.

Baor, L. and I. Blickstein 2005. En route to an "instant family": psychosocial considerations. *Obstet Gynecol Clin North Am.* 32(1): 127-39.

Boivin, Jacky with Bunting Laura, Collins John A. and. Nygren Karl G. 2007. NEW DEBATE. International estimates of infertility prevalence and treatment-seeking: potential need and demand for infertility medical care, *Human Reproduction*, 22 (6): 1506-1512.

Broekmans, F.J. with J. Kwee, D.J. Hendriks, B.W. Mol and C.B. Lambalk 2006. A systematic review of tests predicting ovarian reserve and IVF outcome, *Hum Reprod Update*, 12: 685-718.

Cocksedge, K.A. with T.C. Li, S.H. Saravelos, M. Metwally 2008. A reappraisal of the role of polycystic ovary syndrome in recurrent miscarriage. *Reprod*. 17(1): 151-160.

Dam, P. with H.H. Shirazee, S.K. Goswami, S. Ghosh, A. Ganesh, K. Chaudhury and B. Chakravarty 2006. Role of latent genital tuberculosis in repeated IVF failure in the Indian clinical setting, *Gynecol Obstet Invest*. 61(4): 223-7.

den Hartog, J.E. with C.M. Lardenoije, J.L. Severens, J.A. Land, J.L. Evers and A.G. Kessels 2008. Screening strategies for tubal factor sub-fertility, *Hum Reprod*, 23: 1840-1848.

de Kretser, D.M. 1997. Male infertility, *Lancet*, 349: 787-790.

Diamanti-Kandarakis, E. and A. Dunaif 1996. New perspectives in polycystic ovary syndrome, *Trends Endocrinol Metab* 7(8): 267-271.

Dicker, D. with J.A. Goldman, J. Ashkenazi , D. Feldberg , M. Shelef and T. Levy 1991. Age and pregnancy rates in vitro fertilization, *J., In Vitro Fert Embryo Transf.* 8(3): 141-144.

Evers, J.L. 2002. Female sub-fertility, *Lancet*. 360: 151-159.

Gleicher, N. and D. Barad 2006. An evolutionary concept of polycystic ovarian disease: does evolution favour reproductive success over survival? *Reprod Biomed Online* 12(5):587-9.

Gougeon, A. 1996. Regulation of ovarian follicular development in primates: facts and hypotheses, *Endocr Rev* 17:121-155.

Gunnell, D.J. and P. Ewings 1994. Infertility prevalence, needs assessment and purchasing, *J. Public Health Med.* 16:29-35.

Hart, R.2008. PCOS and infertility, *Panminerva Med*. 50(4): 305-14.

Hunault, C.C. with J.S. Laven, I. van Rooij, M.J. Eijkemans, E.R. te Velde, and J.D. Habbema 2005. Prospective validation of two models predicting pregnancy leading to live birth among untreated sub-fertile couples, *Hum Reprod*. 20: 1636-1641.

Hull, M.G. with C.M. Glazener, N.J. Kelly, D.I. Conway, P.A. Foster, R.A. Hinton, C. Coulson, P.A. Lambert, E.M. Watt and K.M. Desai 1985. Population study of causes, treatment, and outcome of infertility, *Br Med J.* 291:1693-1697.

Inhorn, M.C. 2003. Global infertility and the globalization of new reproductive technologies: illustrations from Egypt, *Soc Sci Med* 56(9): 1837-51.

Jones, Roger (ed.) 2005. *905 Oxford Textbook of Primary Medical Care Vol. 2: Clinical Management,* Oxford: Oxford University Press.

Jorgensen, N. with E. Carlsen, I. Nermoen, M. Punab, J. Suominen, A.G. Andersen, A.M. Andersson, T.B. Haugen, A. Horte and T.K. Jensen 2002. East-West gradient in semen quality in the Nordic–Baltic area: a study of men from the general population in Denmark, Norway, Estonia and Finland, *Human Reproduction* 17: 2199-2208.

Kailasam, C. with S.D. Keay, P. Wilson, W.C. Ford and J.M. Jenkins 2004. Defining poor ovarian response during IVF cycles, in women aged <40 years, and its relationship with treatment outcome, *Hum Reprod*, 19:1544-1547.

Klinkert, E.R. with F.J. Broekmans, C.W. Looman and E.R. te Velde 2004. A poor response in the first in-vitro fertilization cycle is not necessarily related to a poor prognosis in subsequent cycles, *Fertil Steril* 81:1247-1253.

Klinkert, E.R. with F.J. Broekmans, C.W. Looman, J.D. Habbema and E.R. te Velde 2005. Expected poor responders on the basis of an antral follicle count do not benefit from a higher starting dose of gonadotrophins in IVF treatment: a randomized controlled trial. *Hum Reprod*, 20:611-615.

Larsen, U. 2005. Research on infertility: which definition should we use? *Fertil Steril* 83:846-852.

Loutradi, K.E. with E.M. Kolibianakis, C.A. Venetis, E.G. Papanikolaou, G. Pados, I. Bontis and B.C. Tarlatzis 2008. Cryopreservation of human embryos by vitrification or slow freezing: a systematic review and meta-analysis, *Fertil Steril* 90: 186-193.

Macaluso, M. with T.J. Wright-Schnapp, A. Chandra, R. Johnson, C.L. Satterwhite, A. Pulver S.M. Berman, R.Y. Wang, S.L. Farr and L.A. Pollack 2010. A public health focus on infertility prevention, detection, and management, *Fertil Steril* 93(1):16.e1-10.

National Institute for Clinical Excellence 2004. Clinical Guideline 11. Fertility: Assessment and Treatment for People with Fertility Problems. Electronic document,http://www.nice.org.uk/nicemedia/pdf CG011 niceguideline.pdf. Accessed February 1, 2005.

Ombelet, W. with I. Cooke, S. Dyer, G. Serour and P. Devroey 2008. Infertility and the provision of infertility medical services in developing countries, *Hum Reprod Update* 14(6): 605-621.

Ozkans Mur K.W. and A. Arici 2008. Endometriosis and infertility, epidemiology and evidence-based treatments, *Ann N Y Acad Sci* 1127:92-100.

Parikh, F.R. with S.G. Nadkarni, S.A. Kamat, N. Naik, S.B. Soonawala and R.M. Parikh 1997. Genital tuberculosis—a major pelvic factor causing infertility in Indian women, *Fertil Steril* 67(3): 497-500.

Schmidt, L. 2006. Infertility and assisted reproduction in Denmark: Epidemiology and psycho-social consequences, *Dan Med Bull.*53(4): 390-417.

Singh, N. with G. Sumana, S. Mital 2008. Genital tuberculosis: a leading cause for infertility in women seeking assisted conception in North India, *Arch Gynecol Obstet* 278: 325-327.

Spira, A. 1986. Epidemiology of human reproduction, *Hum Reprod* 1: 111-115.

Stephen, E.H. and A. Chandra 2006. Declining estimates of infertility in the United States: 1982-2002, *Fertil Steri* 86:516-523.

Tarlatzis, B.C. with L. Zepiridi, G. Grimbizis and J. Bontis 2003. Clinical management of low ovarian response to stimulation for IVF: a systematic review, *Hum Reprod Update* 9: 61-76.

Trounson, A.O. 1993. IVF and related technology: The present and the future, *Med J Aust* 158 (12): 853-857.

Tsarev, I. with V. Gagonin, A. Giwercman and J. Erenpreiss 2005. Sperm concentration in Latvian military conscripts as compared with other countries in the Nordic–Baltic area, *Int J Androl* 28: 208-214.

Unisa, S. 1999. Childlessness in Andhra Pradesh, India: treatment-seeking and consequences, *Reprod Health Matter* 7: 54-64.

Vayena, E. with P.J. Rowe and P.D. Griffin. 2001. *Medical, ethical and social aspects of assisted reproduction. Current practices and controversies in assisted reproduction:* Report of a WHO meeting, Geneva, Switzerland.

Visser, L. and S. Repping 2010. Unravelling the genetics of spermatogenic failure, *Reproduction* 139: 303-307.

World Health Organization 1999. *WHO Laboratory Manual for the Examination of Human Semen and Sperm-cervical Mucus Interaction. 4th ed.* Cambridge: Cambridge University Press.

World Health Organization 2000. *WHO manual for the standardised investigation and diagnosis of infertile couple,* Cambridge: Cambridge University Press.

Youssry, M. with B. Ozmen, K. Zohni, K. Diedrich and S. Al-Hasani 2008. Current aspects of blastocyst cryopreservation, *Reprod Biomed Online* 16: 311-320.

Zarger, A.H. with A.I. Wani, S.R. Masoodi *et al.* 1997. Epidemiologic and etiologic aspects of primary infertility in the Kashmir region of India, *Fertil Steril* 68:637-43.

Zegers-Hochschild, F. with K.G. Nygren, D. Adamson, J. de Mouzon, P. Lancaster, R. Mansour and E. Sullivan 2006. The International Committee Monitoring Assisted Reproductive Technologies (ICMART) glossary on ART terminology, *Fertility and Sterility* 86 (1):16-19.

19

Pattern of Adolescent Growth Among the Bhotia Boys

Chittaranjan Mandal

Introduction

Growth is the biological synthesis of living tissues and largely attributed by the multiplication of cells. Differential growth rates vary from one part of the body to another and one tissue to another. Adolescence is a period of rapid accretion of new tissue and other widespread developmental changes which are accompanied by increased nutritional requirements relative to the childhood years.

The principal changes that occur during the period of adolescent growth or onset of puberty are detailed by Marshall and Tanner (1986), which are as follows:

1. The adolescent growth spurt, i.e., an acceleration followed by declaration of growth in most skeletal dimensions and in many internal organs.
2. The development of gonads.
3. The development of the secondary reproductive organs and the secondary sex characters.
4. Changes in body composition i.e., in the quantity and distribution of fat in association with growth of the skeletal and musculature.
5. Development of circulatory and respiratory system leading, particularly in boys, to an increase in strength and endurance.

To evaluate the adolescent growth a cross-sectional study was undertaken among the Bhotia boys of Chamoli district, Uttaranchal, India.

Area and People

The Bhotia boys of Chamoli district of Uttaranchal were selected for the present study. The Bhotias are a tribal population, with Mongoloid morphological features who speak Tibeto-Burman family of languages. The word Bhotia is a generic term for several groups of people inhabiting the ranges along the snowy peaks of the Himalayas. Etymologically, the word Bhotia is popularly believed to have originated from the term *bhot* or more correctly *bod* which means Tibet (Walton 1911).

In Uttaranchal, the Bhotia are one of the earliest inhabitants of the Kumaon and Garhwal hills. They consume large quantities of rice, wheat and pulses. Consumption of meat, milk and milk products is low. The Bhotia are divided into eight Sub-Groups on the basis of religious practices, Territory, occupation and dialect. The Sub-Groups are: (1) Jad, (2) Tolchha, (3) Marchha, (4) Johari, (5) Jethora, (6) Darmi, (7) Chaudansi, and (8) Byansi. The Bhotia practice endogamy at the territorial level and exogamy at the clan/lineage level. The present data were collected on 'Tolchha' and 'Marchha' in and around towns of Joshimath and Gopeshwar of district Chamoli in Uttaranchal.

Methods

Data for the present study were collected from 282 males, ranging in age from 11+ to 17+ years, by cross-sectional method. Measurements were obtained in accordance with the techniques recommended by Martin and Seller (1957). The study area is located 6000 ft. above the sea level. Date of birth of each subject was obtained from school registers/birth certificates. Age was calculated as per decimal calendar. Parent's occupation, income, education etc. were obtained from school records and enquiring from subjects. Maturational indicators like adult voice, facial hair, axial hair and pubic hair were recorded by *status quo* method. Subjects were asked about presence or absence of the indicators. Statistical analysis was performed with the help of SPSS 12.0 for windows.

Results

Table 19.1 details the distribution of boys in different age groups along with average age, its standard deviation and standard error. The average age in all age groups studied nears the mid-point of age groups. S.D. values range from 0.27 to 0.32.

Table 19.1: Distribution of Boys according to Different Age Groups

Age groups	*No.*	*Mean*	*S.D.*	*S.E.*	*Minimum*	*Maximum*
11	40	11.43	0.28	0.045	11.02	11.99
12	40	12.47	0.29	0.05	12.03	12.99
13	40	13.51	0.28	0.04	13.08	13.97
14	41	14.44	0.32	0.05	14.01	14.96
15	40	15.56	0.277	0.04	15.05	15.96
16	40	16.55	0.31	0.05	16.04	16.88
17	41	17.57	0.28	0.04	17.01	17.95

Maturational indicators were recorded by *status quo* method. Accordingly frequency distributions were calculated at each age group and are reported in Table 19.2 along with median age. 90-95 per cent of the students had reported presence of all maturational indicators by the age of 15 years, except for facial hairs which were present in 87.5 per cent of the subjects. Appearance of pubic hair appears to be the first adolescent event with median age of 13.9 years. Axial hairs were attained at the age of 14 years, whereas facial hairs were the last to appear i.e. at the age of 14.2 years.

Table 19.2: Frequency Distribution of Maturational Indicators on the Basis of Median-age of Bhotia Boys

Age groups	*Number*	*Adult voice*		*Facial hair*		*Axial hair*		*Pubic hair*	
		No.	*%*	*No.*	*%*	*No.*	*%*	*No.*	*%*
11	40	3	7.5	0	0	0	0	0	0
12	40	25	62.5	2	5	2	5	2	5
13	40	31	77.5	8	20	8	20	8	20
14	41	40	97.6	19	46.3	20	48.8	20	48.8
15	40	38	95	35	87.5	36	90	36	90
16	40	40	100	37	92.5	38	95	39	97.5
17	41	41	100	40	97.6	41	100	41	100
Median age			12.2		14.2		14		13.9

Table 19.3: Mean, S.D. and per annum Growth (in %) in Different Measurements

Measurements		*Age Group*						
		11	*12*	*13*	*14*	*15*	*16*	*17*
Weight	Mean	26.09	31.50	35.17	41.54	46.50	49.94	53.30
	S.D.	3.40	5.61	5.97	6.07	7.10	7.00	5.61
	PAG (%)		20.74	11.65	18.11	11.94	7.40	6.73
Height	Mean	130.11	138.66	145.57	155.12	158.84	161.87	164.19
	S.D.	5.54	6.45	7.77	6.44	8.65	5.54	4.86
	PAG (%)		6.57	4.98	6.56	2.40	1.91	1.43
Sitting height	Mean	69.51	73.19	76.84	81.25	83.61	85.51	86.63
	S.D.	2.33	3.60	4.24	4.30	4.44	3.53	3.00
	PAG (%)		5.29	4.99	5.74	2.90	2.27	1.31
Total arm length	Mean	55.88	59.75	62.49	67.20	68.69	70.05	70.92
	S.D.	2.79	3.26	3.55	2.68	3.91	2.69	2.46
	PAG (%)		6.92	4.58	7.54	2.22	1.97	1.24
Leg length	Mean	60.61	65.46	68.73	73.87	75.22	76.36	77.55
	S.D.	4.06	3.83	4.51	3.00	4.78	3.42	3.90
	PAG (%)		8.00	4.99	7.48	1.83	1.51	1.56
Biacromial diameter	Mean	28.51	30.56	32.03	34.02	35.90	36.67	37.18
	S.D.	1.33	1.52	2.10	2.88	2.59	2.21	1.59
	PAG (%)		7.19	4.81	6.21	5.53	2.14	1.39
Bi-illiocristal diameter	Mean	19.82	20.80	21.76	22.97	23.97	24.18	25.05
	S.D.	1.08	1.58	1.64	1.58	1.83	1.57	1.56
	PAG (%)		4.94	4.61	5.56	4.35	0.88	3.60
Neck circumference	Mean	26.26	27.60	28.37	30.08	31.88	32.55	33.31
	S.D.	1.00	1.48	1.67	1.84	1.76	1.95	1.42
	PAG (%)		5.10	2.79	6.03	5.98	2.10	2.33
Chest circumference	Mean	61.88	66.35	68.52	73.17	77.52	79.45	81.76
	S.D.	3.48	5.23	4.59	5.84	5.21	5.29	4.13
	PAG (%)		7.22	3.27	6.78	5.94	2.49	2.91
M.U.A.C.	Mean	16.95	18.58	19.22	20.63	22.28	23.00	23.88
	S.D.	1.48	2.07	1.93	1.93	2.62	1.88	1.80
	PAG (%)		9.62	3.44	7.34	8.00	3.23	3.83
Calf circumference	Mean	24.74	26.99	27.96	29.74	31.177	31.76	32.10
	S.D.	1.58	2.18	2.21	2.10	2.14	2.19	1.81
	PAG (%)		9.09	3.59	6.37	4.81	1.89	1.07
Tricep skin fold	Mean	5.79	6.14	5.97	5.48	5.33	5.40	5.85
	S.D.	1.71	2.63	2.01	1.59	1.29	1.66	2.16
	PAG (%)		6.04	-2.77	-8.21	-2.74	1.31	8.33

Anthropometric measurements are presented in Table 19.3, while distance curves of different measurements are presented in Figure 19.1 and velocity curves are shown in Figure 19.2.

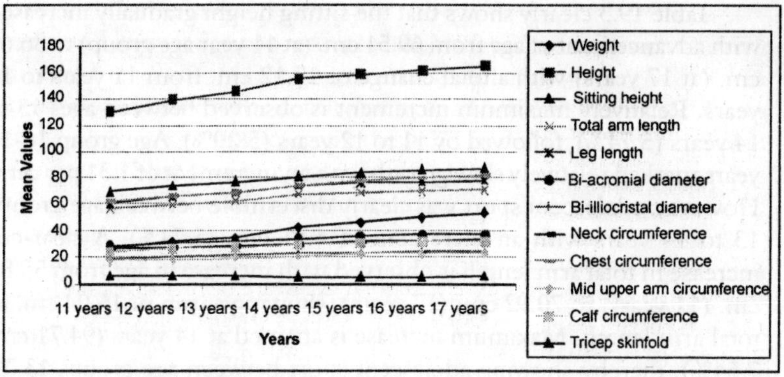

Fig. 19.1: Distance Curve

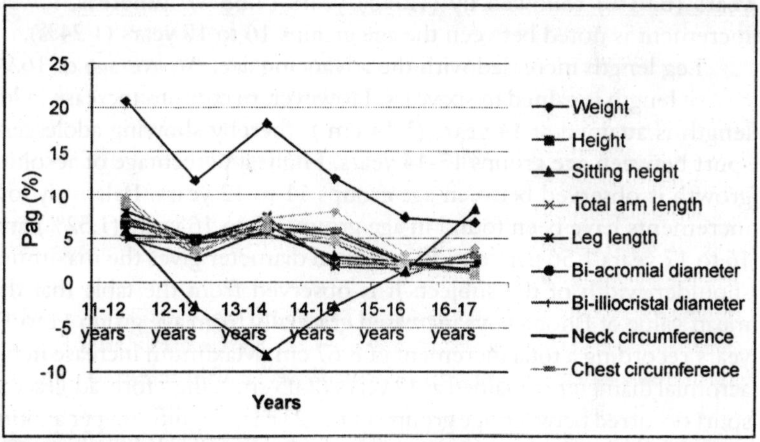

Fig. 19.2: Velocity Curve

Weight increased with the advancing age. An average of 27.21 kg. of weight was gained in six years from 11-17 years. However, maximum increase in weight was attained at 14 years (6.37 kg), thereby showing adolescent spurt between age groups 13-14 years, followed by a relatively low increment at 16 years (3.44 kg.) and 17 years (3.36 kg) age groups. Like body weight stature also increased gradually with the advancing age. Initially rapid increment of height was gained between age groups 11-12 (6.57%) and followed by 13-14 (6.56%) years. On the other hand relatively lowest increment of height was gained between age groups 16 to 17 years (1.43%). Adolescent spurt occurred between 13-14 years with per annum change of 9.55 cm.

Table 19.3 clearly shows that the sitting height gradually increased with advancement of age from 69.51 cm. (at 11 year age group) to 86.63 cm. (at 17 years) with a total change of 17.12 cm. from 11 years to 17 years. Relatively maximum increment is observed between ages 13 to 14 years (5.74%), followed by 11 to 12 years (5.29%). Age group 16-17 years marked relatively slow growth with an increment of 1.31 per cent. However, adolescent spurt was clearly discernible between age groups 13 to 14 years with an increment of 4.41 cm. (5.74%). A clear-cut increase in total arm length is observed with increase in age from 55.88 cm. (11 years) to 70.92 cm. (17 years), showing a gain of 15.04 cm. in total arm length. Maximum increase is attained at 14 years (94.71 cm; 7.54%), thereby showing adolescent spurt between age groups 13-14 years. Next highest increment is recorded between age groups 11-12 years (6.91%) followed by (12-13) years (4.58%). Whereas, lowest increment is noted between the age groups 16 to 17 years (1.24%).

Leg length increased with the advancing age. An average of 16.94 cm. of length is gained in six years. However, maximum increase in leg length is attained at 14 years (5.14 cm.), thereby showing adolescent spurt between age groups 13-14 years. Highest percentage of absolute growth is observed between age groups 11 to 12 years. Relatively low increments have been found in age groups 15 to 16 years (1.52%) and 16 to 17 years 1.56 per cent. Bi-acromial diameter gives the maximum shoulder width of the subject. It is observed from the table that the mean value of Bhotia boys increased gradually from age group 11 to 17 years recording a total increment of 8.67 cm. Maximum increase in bi-acromial diameter is attained at 12 years (2.05 cm.), therefore, adolescent spurt occurred between age groups 11 to 12 years. Significant per annum growth occurred up to 15 years of age. Bi-illiocristal diameter gives maximum width of the pelvis. Like shoulder width, bi-illiocristal diameter recorded gradual increment in average values up to age group 17 years, with a total increment of 5.23 cm. Maximum increase in bi-illiocristal diameter is attained at 14 years (1.21 cm.; 5.5%), thereby showing adolescent spurt between age groups 13 to 14 years.

It revealed that neck circumference increased gradually from age group 11 to 17 years recording a total increment of 7.05 cm. Maximum per annum growth is recorded between age groups 14 to 15 years (1.80 cm.), showing adolescent spurt. Chest circumference recorded a total average gain of 19.88 cm. with gradual increase in chest dimensions with growing age. Maximum increment is recorded at age group 14 years (4.65 cm.), thereby reflecting adolescent spurt between age groups

13 to 14 years. However, significant inter age group changes are recorded from 11 to 15 years and thereafter 16 to 17 years. It is observed from the Table that mid-upper arm circumference increased with growing age with a total average increment of 6.93 cm. from 11 to 17 years. Maximum increment is recorded between age groups 14 to 15 years (1.65 cm). Like other parameters, calf circumference increased with increase in age with a total average increment of 7.36 cm. Maximum increase in calf circumference is attained at 12 years (2.25 cm.), thereby showing adolescent spurt between age groups 11 to 12 years. Thereafter, though the average measurements increased but tempo of increment fluctuated.

The mean values of Triceps Skinfold thickness fluctuated with growing age. It recorded slight increment between age groups 11 to 12 years. For next three years a decrease in skinfold measurements is found, which is more marked between the age groups 13-14 years. The skinfold thickness at triceps again showed increase in following years i.e., from 16 to 17 years with maximum per annum increment between age groups 16-17 years (8.33%).

In Table 19.4 the degree of concomitant variation (or co-variation) between two variables is furnished. Coefficient of correlation values are calculated between all the measurements. Values are invariably significant for all possible combinations. However, only some selected correlation values are depicted in Table 19.4.

Discussion

It can be seen from various observations that there is often a variation in the tempo of growth in different body-parts. Externally this means that human body is continuously changing its size and shape. The variation of the speed of growth between one body part and another is regulated, so that each part reaches its size, proportional to the role it has to play in the body's physiology at the correct time. The children for the present study invariably are from families of agriculturist, and belong to nuclear families. Majority of the students come from medium size family (i.e., 4-6 members). In most of the cases (61.70%), family income is invariably between Rs. 1,000 to Rs. 4,999 p.m. (i.e., lower income group). 17.38 per cent of fathers were illiterate and 8.86 per cent of father had graduate level of education. On the other hand 39.36 per cent of the subjects have illiterate mothers also. The analysis of different measurements clearly point to the adolescent spurt at age

Table 19.4: Correlation Coefficient among some Measurements

Correlations	*Age groups*						
	11	12	13	14	15	16	17
Height *vs.* weight	0.791	0.653	0.852	0.818	0.82	0.676	0.528
Height *vs.* Sitting height	0.759	0.86	0.881	0.92	0.933	0.804	0.598
Bi-acromial diameter *vs.* Bi-illiocristal diameter	0.499	0.694	0.664	0.486	0.648	0.589	0.068
Total arm length *vs.* Stature	0.867	0.912	0.895	0.873	0.911	0.807	0.71
Tr. Skinfold *vs.* M.U.A.C.	0.671	0.701	0.427	0.372	0.469	0.284	0.462
M.U.A.C. *vs.* Total arm length	0.537	0.361	0.626	0.682	0.371	0.375	-0.274
Height *vs.* Calf cir.	0.62	0.637	0.764	0.656	0.666	0.505	0.302

Table 19.5: Comparison of Growth among Bhotia and Garhwali Boys

Measurements		AGE GROUP 11		12		13		14		15		16		17	
		Bhotia (n = 40)	Garhwali Rajputs (n = 42)	Bhotia (n = 40)	Garhwali Rajputs (n = 46)	Bhotia (n = 40)	Garhwali Rajputs (n = 49)	Bhotia (n = 41)	Garhwali Rajputs (n = 47)	Bhotia (n = 40)	Garhwali Rajputs (n = 45)	Bhotia (n = 40)	Garhwali Rajputs (n = 47)	Bhotia (n = 41)	Garhwali Rajputs (n = 40)
Weight	1	26.09	31.3	31.50	35.13	35.17	39.60	41.54	42.70	46.50	47.60	49.94	49.06	53.30	50.86
	2	0.54	0.85	0.89	0.82	0.94	1.04	0.95	1.05	1.12	1.16	1.11	1.17	0.88	1.20
Height	1	130.11	139.61	138.66	146.48	145.57	154.91	155.12	158.89	158.84	165.70	161.87	164.87	164.19	165.89
	2	0.88	1.21	1.02	1.40	1.23	1.32	1.01	1.22	1.37	1.24	0.88	1.02	0.76	0.97
Sitting height	1	69.51	72.43	73.19	75.87	76.84	79.10	81.25	81.96	83.61	85.60	85.51	85.37	86.63	86.43
	2	0.37	0.56	0.57	0.79	0.67	0.79	0.67	0.68	0.70	0.66	0.56	0.60	0.47	0.49
Total arm length	1	55.88	59.90	59.75	63.15	62.49	67.83	67.20	69.02	68.69	71.80	70.05	71.57	70.92	72.84
	2	0.44	0.57	0.52	0.68	0.56	0.72	0.42	0.62	0.62	0.56	0.43	0.53	0.38	0.62
Leg length	1	60.611	67.17	65.46	70.60	68.73	75.81	73.87	76.92	75.22	80.14	76.36	79.50	77.55	79.20
	2	0.64	0.76	0.61	1.00	0.71	0.74	0.47	0.70	0.76	0.72	0.54	0.75	0.61	0.68
Biacromial diameter	1	28.51	30.63	30.56	32.11	32.03	33.67	34.02	34.69	35.90	36.50	36.67	36.81	37.18	37.63
	2	0.21	0.40	0.24	0.34	0.33	0.40	0.45	0.37	0.41	0.41	0.35	0.34	0.25	0.40
Bi-illiocristal diameter	1	19.82	22.22	20.80	23.40	21.76	24.62	22.97	25.08	23.97	26.30	24.18	26.22	25.05	26.65
	2	0.17	0.23	0.25	0.22	0.26	0.48	0.25	0.26	0.29	0.32	0.25	0.26	0.24	0.24
Neck circumference	1	26.26	27.36	27.60	27.47	28.37	29.07	30.08	30.20	31.88	31.20	32.55	31.81	33.31	32.35
	2	0.16	0.29	0.23	0.39	0.26	0.25	0.29	0.29	0.28	0.30	0.31	0.30	0.22	0.31
Chest circumference	1	61.88	63.75	66.35	66.31	68.52	69.36	73.17	71.83	77.52	74.43	79.45	75.91	81.76	76.69
	2	0.55	0.61	0.83	0.70	0.73	0.63	0.91	0.71	0.82	0.78	0.84	0.86	0.65	0.80
MUAC	1	16.95	17.86	18.58	19.02	19.22	19.47	20.63	20.10	22.28	21.20	23.00	21.58	23.88	21.99
	2	0.24	0.24	0.33	0.31	0.31	0.26	0.30	0.29	0.41	0.31	0.30	0.34	0.28	0.30
Calf circumference	1	24.74	26.29	26.99	27.93	27.96	29.21	29.74	30.13	31.17	30.74	31.76	30.91	32.10	31.02
	2	0.25	0.35	0.35	0.35	0.35	0.33	0.33	0.34	0.34	0.30	0.35	0.40	0.28	0.45
Tricep skinfold	1	5.79	7.61	6.14	7.66	5.97	6.89	5.48	6.88	5.33	7.02	5.40	7.05	5.85	7.78
	2	0.27	0.28	0.42	0.49	0.32	0.30	0.25	0.35	0.20	0.37	0.26	0.51	0.34	0.54
BMI	1	15.36	15.91	16.32	16.30	16.49	16.40	17.18	16.80	18.33	17.28	19.00	17.94	19.76	18.42
	2	0.20	0.26	0.35	0.24	0.25	0.25	0.25	0.30	0.27	0.33	0.33	0.26	0.27	0.34

Note: 1 = Mean; 2 = S.E. of mean

Table 19.6: Comparison of Weight among Different Populations

Age group	Bhotia	NCHS 1966-70	ICMR	ICMR U.P.	Garhwali Rajputs	Garhwali Brahmins
11	26.09	38.4	25.9	26.3	31.26	31.22
12	31.5	42.98	28.5	28.8	35.13	34.48
13	35.17	50	32.1	32.6	39.6	38.93
14	41.54	56.66	35.7	36.6	42.7	42.81
15	46.5	61.61	39.6	41	47.6	45.33
16	49.94	64.82	43.2	44.3	49.06	49.7
17	53.3	68.03	45.7	46.2	50.86	51.05

Table 19.7: Comparison of Height among Different Populations

Age group	Bhotia	NCSH 1966-70	ICMR	ICMR U.P.	Garhwali Rajputs	Garhwali Brahmins
11	130.11	145.7	133.4	132.8	139.61	140.37
12	138.66	152.3	138.3	137.8	146.48	147.91
13	145.57	159.8	144.6	145.1	154.91	154.28
14	155.12	166.7	150.1	150.8	158.89	160.15
15	158.84	171.4	155.5	157.1	165.7	163.95
16	161.87	174.3	159.5	160.0	164.87	166.51
17	164.19	175.5	161.4	160.6	165.89	166.79

groups 13-14 years in most of the measurements. Bi-acromial diameter and calf circumference attain peak velocity between age groups 11-12 years. Triceps skinfold, decreased in fat deposit from age group 12-13 years, and gradually increase to attain peak values at age group 17 years. Values of Body Mass Index increase with advancing age, which record peak increments between age groups 14-15 years.

Comparison of all anthropometric parameters of the present study with the Garhwali Rajput Boys (Kaul and Tandon 2001: Table 19.5) studied in Dehradun show that in case of Height, Total arm length, Leg length, Bi-acromial breadth, Bi-cristal breadth and Tricep Skinfold, the Garhwali Rajput boys have greater dimensions than Bhotia boys at all age groups. Same trend is found for sitting height, except at 16 years, where Bhotias show greater measurements. Weight and calf circumference are greater among the Garhwali Rajputs from 11-14 years, whereas mid-upper arm circumference show greater dimensions up to 13 years and thereafter Bhotia attain higher mean values. Neck and chest circumference are greater in Bhotias, except at 13 years for both measurements and in addition at 14 years for neck circumference. Except at 11 years, Bhotia have higher mean values for BMI, than

Garhwali Rajput at all age groups, thereby showing proportionately higher weight. The adolescent spurt occurred between the ages 13-14 years among Bhotias in most of the measurements, which is one year prior to that found among Garhwali Rajputs (i.e., 14-15 years).

The growth data have also been compared with NCHS Standards (1966-70), ICMR Standards (1972), ICMR U.P. data (1972), based on data collected during 1956-1966 and Garhwali Brahmin populations of Dehradun (Tandon and Kaul 2003) in Tables 19.6 and 19.7 and depicted in Figures 19.3 and 19.4. The weight and height of Bhotia boys are below the NCHS standards at all ages. Bhotia boys invariably have more weight and height than ICMR standards and ICMR U.P. data at all age groups, except in the weight of ICMR U.P. data and in the height of ICMR standard and ICMR U.P. data at 11 years age group

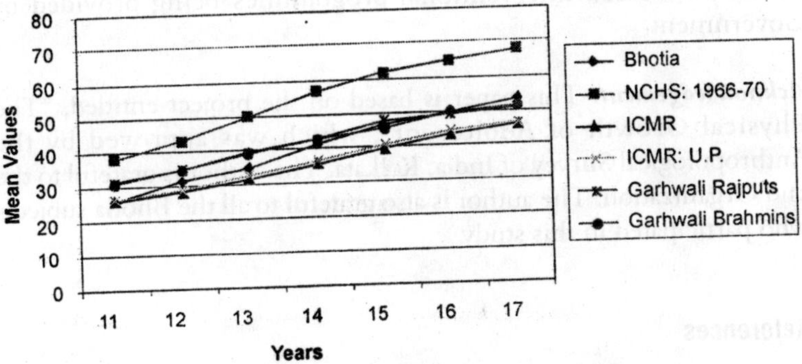

Fig. 19.3: Comparison of Weight among Different Populations

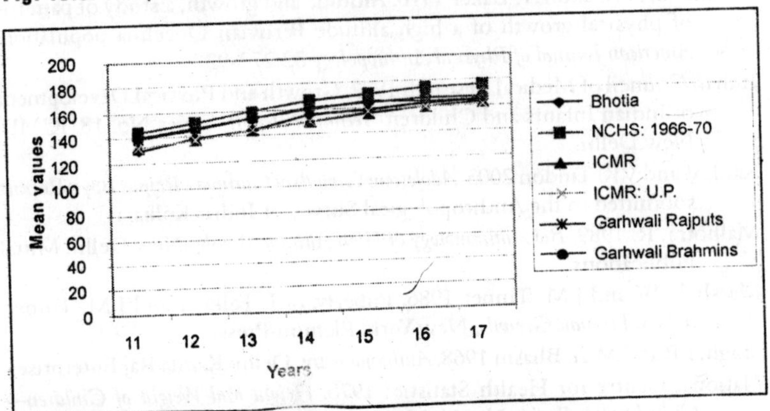

Fig. 19.4: Comparison of Height among Different Populations

only. Up to 14 years of age, Garhwali Brahmins are heavier than the Bhotia, thereafter, the Bhotia outweigh the Garhwali Brahmins. So far height is concerned, the Garhwali Brahmins are taller than Bhotias at all age groups.

It can be inferred from the comparative analysis of Bhotias and other populations that Bhotias, Garhwali Rajputs and Garhwali Brahmins exhibit some differences in their pattern of growth. It may further be stated that these differences, may be attributed to genetic variation, differences in demographic parameters and due to differences of altitudinal zone. All these points were also supported by the previous studies (Frisancho and Baker 1970, Malhotra 1989, Singh and Nath 1997). The well off conditions of the present sample than ICMR standards and ICMR U.P. data, can be explained due to comparatively good environmental conditions, medium size family, besides increased interventional programmes being provided by Government.

Acknowledgement: This paper is based on the project entitled, "The Physical Growth of Adolescent", which was approved by the Anthropological Survey of India, Kolkata. The author is grateful to the said Organization. The author is also grateful to all the Bhotia subjects who participated in this study.

References

Frisancho, A.R. and P.T. Baker 1970. Altitude and growth, a study of patterns of physical growth of a high altitude Peruvian Quechua population, *American Journal of Physical Anthropology* 32:272-92.

Indian Council of Medical Research 1972. Growth and Physical Development of Indian Infants and Children. *Technical Report*, Series No. 18. ICMR, New Delhi.

Kaul, V. and V.K. Tandon 2003. *Adolescent Growth of Garhwali Rajput Boys*. Report submitted to the Anthropological Survey of India: Kolkata.

Malhotra, R. 1989. *Bio Anthropology of High Altitude People*, New Delhi: Mittal Publications.

Marshall, W. and J.M. Tanner 1986. Puberty, *In* F. Falkner and J.M. Tanner. (eds.). *Human Growth*, New York: Plenum Press.

Singh, I.P. and M.K. Bhasin 1968. *Anthropometry*, Delhi: Kamla Raj Enterprises.

National Centre for Health Statistics 1970. *Height and Weight of Children—United States.* Series No. 11, No. 104 (Children aged 6 years to 11 years).

U.S. Department of Health, Education and Welfare Public Health Services.

Singh, R. and S. Nath 1997. Comparative Growth Patterns among the Jatav and Chauhan males of district Moradabad, U.P., *Journal of Anthropological Survey of India*. 46(1): 69-77.

Singh, K.S. 1994. *People of India. The Schedule Tribes*. National Series, Vol. III, Anthropological Survey of India, Kolkata, Delhi: Oxford University Press.

WHO 1995. *The use and interpretation of anthropometry*. Report of WHO Expert Committee, Geneva. WHO Technical Report Series, 854.

20

Trepanation: A Surgical Operation Practiced in Prehistoric Society

Jhillika Paul

Introduction

Anthropologists often obtain data on health, disease and death from ancient populations using the methods of palaeopathology, the study of ancient diseases. The primary source of palaeopathological information is skeletal remains. Archaeologists increasingly use palaeopathology as an important main tool for understanding the lives of ancient peoples. Evidence for trepanation is also common. Skulls with multiple holes show that some patients survived this procedure many times, because the bone has begun the knit back together. Trepanation (also known as trepanning, trephination, trephining or making a burr hole) is a medical intervention in which a hole is drilled or scrapped into the human skull, in order to treat health problems related to intracranial diseases. Evidence of trepanation has been found in prehistoric human remains from Neolithic times onwards. People believed the practice would cure epileptic seizures, migraines, and mental disorders. The bone that was trepanned was kept by the prehistoric people and probably worn as a charm to keep evil spirits away. Evidence also suggests that trepanation was primitive emergency surgery after head wounds to remove shattered bits of bone from a fractured skull and clean out the blood that often pools under the skull after a blow to the head. Such injuries were typical for primitive weaponry such as slings and war clubs. It may also refer to any "burr" hole created through other body surfaces, including nail beds. It is often used to relieve pressure beneath a surface. A trephine is an instrument used for cutting out a round piece of skull bone. There is some contemporary use of the term. In modern eye surgery a trephine instrument is used in corneal transplant surgery. The procedure of drilling a hole through a fingernail or toenail is also known as trephination. It is performed by a physician or surgeon to relieve the pain mainly. Modern surgeons generally use the term craniotomy for this procedure. The removed piece of skull is typically replaced as soon as possible.

Distribution of Evidences and Procedures

Different diseases and ailments were common in prehistory than are prevalent today; there is evidence that many people suffered from osteoarthritis, probably caused by the lifting of heavy objects which would have been a daily and necessary task in their societies. The transport of, for example, latte stones, involving hyperextension and torque of the lower back, while dragging the stones, may have contributed to the development of micro fractures in the spine and subsequent spondylolysis. Things such as cuts, bruises and breakages of a bone, without antiseptics, proper facilities or knowledge of germs, would become very serious if infected. There is also evidence of rickets bone deformity and bone wastage (Osteomalacia), which is caused by a lack of Vitamin D.

The life expectancy in prehistoric times was low, 25-40 years with men living longer than women; archaeological evidence of women and babies found together suggests that many women would have died in childbirth, perhaps accounting for the lower life expectancy in women than men. Another possible explanation for the shorter life spans of prehistoric women may be malnutrition; men, as hunters, generally received better food than their female counterparts, who would subsequently have been less resistant to disease.

Prehistoric societies believed in both natural and supernatural means of variably causing and treating disease. For serious or disabling diseases, like epilepsy, migraine, for which there was no rational cause, blame was placed on the supernatural—gods, evil spirits and sorcery. It was believed that evil spirits, conjured by a sorcerer, could inhabit a person's body and cause illness and that these spirits could be removed from the patient, through the skull, by trepanning, and through other treatments carried out by a shaman, a medicine man. Logic and reasoning were used to deduce the cause of injuries. Injuries, for which there was a clear cause, were not blamed on the supernatural.

Plant materials (herbs), earths and clays may have provided prehistoric peoples with some of their first medicines, used for treatments for diseases in prehistoric cultures. Since plant materials quickly rot under most conditions, historians are unlikely to fully understand which species were used in prehistoric medicine. An idea can be obtained by looking at the climate of the respective society and which species continue to grow there today and through anthropological studies of existing indigenous peoples.

Trepanation is perhaps the oldest surgical procedure for which there is evidence, and in some areas may have been quite widespread. Out of 120 prehistoric skulls found at one burial site in France dated to 6500 BC, 40 had trepanation holes. Many prehistoric and pre modern patients had signs of their skull structure healing; suggesting that many of those subjected to the surgery survived, as there is evidence of bone tissue surrounding the surgical hole partially grown back, therefore survival of the procedure did occur. Healing and survival after trepanation suggesting that the survival rate of the operations was high and the infection rate was low. Among New World societies, trepanning is most commonly found in the Andean civilizations such as the pre-Incan culture. The archaeological record in Mesoamerica is further complicated by the practice of skull mutilation and modification which was carried out after the death of the subject, in order to fashion "trophy skulls" and the like of captives and enemies. Specimens identified from the Maya civilization region of southern Mexico, Guatemala and the Yucatan Peninsula show no evidence of the drilling or cutting techniques found in central and highland Mexico.

From the study of the skeletal materials found in the Middle Bronze Age graves at Create and Mycenae, it is possible to identify a number of trepanations mostly performed on the parietal and frontal regions of the cranium (and occasionally on the occipital) (Robert Arnott 1997). A confirmed early chalcolithic trepanation (dated approx. 4000 BC) has recently been identified at Kurucay-Hoyuk in south west Anatolia. Here the skull has three holes, each 0.5 cm in diameter, which may have been made by a drill. Until this recent discovery, the oldest recorded trepanation in the region came from a female skeleton found at Elmali-Karatas and dated approx. 2300 B.C. Excavations at Syria in 1987 and 1990 uncovered two clear examples of trepanations being performed in approx. 1700 B.C. The Middle Bronze Age Aegean trepanations are contemporary with those found in Syria. (Erskin Güleç 1995). For comparative analyses, north western Mongolia, Tuva, Kazakhstan and Altai were also included in this study. The data collected by different authors indicate the sporadic appearance of trepanned skulls in these territories.

Burzahom, a neolithic-chalcolithic site of present day Kashmir Valley, India, denotes the first stage of village growth outside the Harappan distribution zone (Krishnaswami 1962) consists of sequences of two Neolithic levels (Periods I and II) successively followed by megalithic (Period III) and early historical (Period IV) periods. Dwelling pits, dug into the local Karewa deposit, were filled up in Period II and their levelled tops were plastered with mud and sometimes painted with red ochre. In Period II three animal and seven human burials are reported, among the later, five are primary and two secondary but both laid in oval pits dug in the floor of a house and lime plastered inside. Bodies were placed in both embryonic and extended positions for burials. In one case the bones are found treated with red ochre solution, which implies that the burial was opened later for rubbing red ochre on the bones of the decomposed body. In this case there are trepanation marks on the skull. The Neolithic skeletons represented long headed skulls and showed dental caries, ante-mortem tooth loss, alveolar abscess, and pulp exposer through attrition. These people of Burzahom have been said to represent a long headed or dolichocranial population of tall to medium stature (Chakrabarti 2006).

It suggests that trepanation might have been practiced in prehistoric India (3000-2800 years ago) for acquired neurological ailments. One female skull from Burzahom, first discovered in 1968, revealed 11 attempts at trephination, with 6 neatly completed circular or oval perforations, all in the left parietal bone. The left calvarium also showed hypertrophy, which could have been related to long-standing atrophy of the underlying brain. It was impossible to establish the precise symptoms that may have afflicted this individual, but the Burzahom female might have been 'insane, epileptic or otherwise different'. The carefully performed trepanation, suggestive of a multistage procedure on a possibly anomalous skull, argues for a surgical approach for medical reasons on a living person. It is also likely that this might have been part of a ritual in a primitive society that regarded epilepsy and other neurological diseases to be a result of demonic possessions (Radhakrishnan 2009).

Evidences are also found from protohistoric societies of India, like in the Harappan Civilisation. At Lothal, Gujarat, a skull of a child attributed a hole on its right temporal bone. According to Roy Chowdhury (1973) the evidence of trepanation was present on Post Harappan skulls No. H 796/B and H 802/B, from Cemetery R37 and on a Kalibangan skull. A megalithic skull (M30) from Maski (Karnataka) in South India also depicts evidence of trepanation with two circular holes respectively on the either side of the sagittal suture of the vertex. (Sarkar 1972).

The common methods for trepanation were: (a) scrapping, (b) grooving, (c) boring and cutting, and (d) rectangular intersecting incisions (Lisowski 1967). The scarpping technique was probably one of the most common methods and was distributed chronologically from ancient Egypt to the Renaissance period in Italy. The grooving technique was also frequently used in many parts of the world and is currently still performed in Kenya. The boring and cutting method was used in Peru. A method in which four straight incisions were made was commonly adopted in Peru, but is also known in Neolithic France, Iron Age Palestine and modern Africa. The classification of trepanation currently in use today includes: (1) Real or surgical trepanation (ante mortem) defined as any opening of the skull on a living person, (2) Ritual trepanation (post mortem) opening with the aim of obtaining a part of the skull vault to be used as amulet or other use (Broca 1877).

The hole or depression in one or both tables of the skull is usually made by scrapping, rasping, and cautery, but may also be accomplished by drilling, boring with a gimlet or knife tip, cutting and sawing. Excavation revealed in a cemetery of Middle Bronze age at Greece a human skeleton with trepanned skull associated with instruments like curved bladed knife, long saw, denticulated forceps, tanged knife, chisels, a long handed spoon or scoop. It is believed some of these used as toilet articles and were adapted for surgical use, as bronze doesn't always produce the most efficient of tools for cutting flesh and bone as it blunts quite easily, knives or scalpels made from a hard stone such as the volcanic glass-obsidian, flint, would have been more in use as surgical instruments (Arnott 1997).

Conclusion

There are several limitations to palaeopathological research. Since skeletal material is the most frequently recovered type of human remains, most palaeopathology studies pertain to diseases that visibly alter or affect bone. Many diseases affect bone in similar ways, thus making it difficult and sometimes impossible to determine the exact disease represented. Many diseases do not affect bone at all, and are only evident in tissue, hair or other rare remains. Palaeopathology currently accounts for only a portion of the total diseases the ravaged past populations. Trephination, although we know very little about the origin of it. Its beginning is not found in rational medical practice. As in ancient societies, it would have made its first appearance in the region as a ritual act and experience would have taught that humans could survive the operation. The operation was probably performed in the hope of curing intracranial disease or extradural haematoma, persistent migraine or paralysis. But it is no more likely that it was a surgical clearing out or the removal of splinters of bone from a head injury brought about by combat, hunting or farming. We cannot rule out however, the possible magical or symbolic use of the operation on the living for the curing of perceived 'mental illness' such as epilepsy or schizophrenia, or for the catharsis of 'evil spirits'. However, it is only possible to speculate as to whether the surgeons in these circumstances had ritual or therapeutic motives.

Though very rare, prehistoric evidences from all-over the world showed trephination as a method of surgery, but some concerning issues like instruments used, specialised executive persons, patient's social status, socio-political background of that society etc. are not clearly revealed and that practice became extinct for successive cultural periods.

References

Arnott, Robert 1997. Surgical Practice in the Prehistoric Aegean, *Medizinhistorisches Journal*, Band 32, Heft 3-4.

Bazarsad, N. and Tumen 1998. Travmaticheskie povrezdeniya na cherepakh Chandmanskogo mogilnika (Traumatic injuries on crania from the Chandman burial ground), *Rossiyskaya Arkheologiya*, 4:122-9.

Broca, P. 1877. Sur la trepanation du crane et les amulettes craniennes a l'epoque neolithique, *Copte rendu du Congres intern. D'Anthropologie et d'Archeologie prehistorique* (On Cranial Trepanation and amulets made from Cranial bone from the Neolithic Period; Proceedings of the International Congress of Prehistoric Anthrology and Archaeology), *1876, Section 8, Vol. I.* Budapest.

Brothwell, Don R. 1963. *Digging up Bones; the Excavation, Treatment and Study of Human Skeletal Remains*. London: British Museum (Natural History).

Chakrabarti, Dilip K. 2006. *The Oxford Companion to Indian Archaeology*, Oxford: Oxford University Press.

Chandy, J. 1954. Surgical Treatment of Epilepsy, *Neurol India* 2: 37-41.

Erskin, Güleç 1995. 'Trepanation in ancient Anatolia: six new case studies' (abstract), *Papers on Paleopathology presented to the 22nd Meeting of the Paleopathology Association, Oakland*, p. 6.

Lisowski, F.P. 1967. Prehistoric and Early Historic Trepanation, *In* D.R. Brothwell and A.T. Sandison (eds.) *Diseases in Antiquity*, Illinois: Charles C. Thomas, pp. 651-72.

Lumholtz, Carl 1897. Trephining in Mexico, *American Anthropologist* 10 (12): 389.

Radhakrishnan, K. 2009. Epilepsy Surgery in India, *Neurol India*, 57:4-6.

Restak, Richard 2000. Fixing the Brain. *Mysteries of the Mind*, National Geographic Society. ISBN 0-792-27941-7OCLC 43662032. Washington, DC.

Schultz, M. 2001. Paleohistopathology of Bone: A New Approach to the Study of Ancient Diseases, *Yearbook of Physical Anthropology*, 44: 106-147.

Stuart, Piggott 1940. A Trepanned Skull of the Beaker Period from Dorset and the Practice of Trepanning in Prehistoric Europe, *Proceedings of the Prehistoric Society*, 6,112-33.

Tiesler Blos, Vera 2003. *Cranial Surgery in Ancient Mesoamerica*. Electronic document, Mesoweb. *http://www.mesoweb.com/features/tiesler/Cranial.pdf*. Accessed March 22, 2010.

21

Automatic Testing for Colour-Blindness

Sandip Dey, Sirsendu Shekhar Ray and *Kaushik Roy*

1. Introduction

Colour-blindness (colour vision deficiency) is a condition in which certain colours cannot be distinguished, and is most commonly due to an inherited condition. Red/Green colour-blindness is by far the most common form, about 99 per cent, and causes problems in distinguishing reds and greens. Another colour deficiency Blue/Yellow also exists, but is rare and there is no commonly available test for it.

Inherited colour blindness is most common, affects both eyes, and does not worsen over time. This type is found in about 8 per cent of males and 0.4 per cent of females. These colour problems are linked to the X chromosome and are almost always passed from a mother to her son.

Colour-blindness may be partial (affecting only some colours), or complete (affecting all colours). Complete colour-blindness is very rare. Those who are completely colour-blind often have other serious eye problems as well.

1.1 Some Major Problems of Colour -Blindness

- Weather forecasts

- Bi-colour and tri-colour LEDs
- Traffic lights, and worst of all, Caution lights
- Colour observation by others
- Purchasing clothing
- Cooking and foods

1.2 Signs and Symptoms

The symptoms of colour blindness are dependent on several factors, such as whether the problem is congenital, acquired, partial, or complete.

- Difficulty distinguishing reds and greens (most common)
- Difficulty distinguishing blues and greens (less common)
- The symptoms of more serious inherited colour vision problems and some types acquired problems may include:
- Objects appear as various shades of gray (this occurs with complete colour-blindness and is very rare)
- Reduced vision
- Nystagmus

1.3 Treatment

There is no treatment or cure for colour-blindness. Those with mild colour deficiencies learn to associate colours with certain objects and are usually able to identify colour as everyone else. However, they are unable to appreciate colour in the same way as those with normal colour vision.

2. Types of Colour-Blindness

There are various types of colour-blindness. They are mainly categorized in two categories:

2.1 Anomalous Trichromacy: A mild shift in the sensitivity of pigments of the cones. It is of three kinds.

2.1.1 Protanomaly (one out of 100 males): Shades of red appear weaker in depth and brightness. Protanomaly is referred to as "red-weakness", an apt description of this form of colour deficiency. Any redness seen in a colour by a normal observer is seen more weakly by the protanomalous viewer, both in terms of its "colouring power" (saturation, or depth of colour) and its brightness.

2.1.2 Deuteranomaly (five out of 100 males): Shades of green appear weaker. Let the deuteranomalous person adjust your television and he would add more green and subtract red. He is considered "green weak". Similar to the protanomalous person, he is poor at discriminating small differences in hues in the red, orange, yellow, green region of the spectrum.

2.1.3 Tritanomaly: Very rare case where shades of blue appear weaker.

2.2 Dichromacy-Great deficiency or missing completely one of the cones. It is of three kinds and it is more common compared to Anomalous Trichromacy. A person with normal colour vision and with Dichromacy type of colour-blindness is shown in Fig. 21.1(a-d).

2.2.1 Protanopia (one out of 100 males): Shades of red are greatly reduced, if present at all, in depth and brightness. For the protanope, the brightness of red, orange, and yellow is much reduced compared to normal. For example *see* Fig. 21.1(b).

2.2.2 Deuteranopia (one out of 100 males): Shades of green are greatly reduced, if present at all, in depth and brightness. The deuteranope suffers the same hue discrimination problems as the protanope, but without the abnormal dimming. For example *see* Fig. 21.1(b).

2.2.3 Tritanopia: Very rare case where shades of blue are greatly reduced, if present at all, in depth and brightness. For example *see* Fig. 21.1(b).

3. What Wavelength Goes with Colour?

Our eyes are sensitive to light which lies in a very small region of the electromagnetic spectrum labelled "visible light". This "visible light" corresponds to a wavelength range of 400-700 nanometers (nm) and a colour range of violet through red. The human eye is not capable of "seeing" radiation with wavelengths outside the visible spectrum. The visible colours from shortest to longest wavelength are: violet, blue, green, yellow, orange, and red. Ultraviolet radiation has a shorter wavelength than the visible violet light. Infrared radiation has a longer wavelength than visible red light. The white light is a mixture of the colours of the visible spectrum. Black is a total absence of light.

Earth's most important energy source is the Sun. Sunlight consists of the entire electromagnetic spectrum. The detailed distribution of such spectrum is shown in Fig. 21.2.

4. Existing Colour-Blindness Test

Ishihara Test: The most famous colour-blindness test was created by Dr. Shinobu Ishihara of University of Tokyo. If we visit an ophthalmologist we will most likely be given some variations of this test.

Waggoner Test: A variant of this test specially designed for pre-school children using shapes instead of numbers has been created and is sold by Dr. Terrace L. Waggoner of the Staff Naval Hospital Pensacola. His site also contains a wealth of general information about colour vision deficiencies.

Yee Test: Arson's friend and collaborator Nick Yee even takes this test a step further on his wave site by including a graphic that reveals one thing to the colour-blind and to those with normal vision. This test does not constitute medical advice.

Clauset Test: This is an unique and very interesting variant to most conventional colour-blind tests has been developed by Aaron Clauset of Haveford College. Unlike most tests, which requires good colour vision, only colour-blind people can pass these tests.

4.1 Limitations of the Existing Models

There are several colour-blindness test model available in the market. All are good in their places. The most common test done for colour-blindness people is Ishihara test. If we visit an ophthalmologist we will most likely be given some variation of this test. Here a man is subjected to some pictures of numbers consisting of dotted pixels of various colours. If he cannot identify it then it proves that he has colour-blindness in some colour.

This test model tells only if a person is colour-blind or not. On the other hand this test is not designed for all categories of man. This test does not tell anything about the band of colours where he/she has colour-blind.

The next test model is Waggoner model. This test model is specially designed for pre-school children using shapes instead of numbers.

In this test model some shapes of different colours comes to the pre-school children and they identify the shapes. If children do not identify shapes, then this proves that the children are colour-blind. This test does not tell anything about the band of colours where he/she has colour-blindness.

The next test model is Clauset Test Model. Unlike most tests, which require good colour vision, only the colour-blind people can pass on this test.

The next test model is Yee test model. Arson's friend and collaborator Nick Yee even takes this test a step further on his website by including a graphic that reveals one thing to the colour-blind and to those with normal vision. This test does not constitute medical advice.

The other entire existing model tests for some categories of people. There is no such common test model, which can test for colour-blindness for all people.

5. Proposed System

The implementation of this proposed system is based on the idea that a colour-blind person can't differentiate between similar colours in which he is colour-blind. For this we have considered digital eight (8). As it consists of 7 lines and depending on absent of one or more lines it is converted into different digits. For example if the middle line is absent it will be zero (0) instead of eight (8). We have carefully designed the lines of this number and also backgrounds of there lines. The various buttons are also designed keeping in mind the possible numbers/shapes will be seen by a colour-blind person. We have taken utmost care to consider all types of possibility in respect to colour-blindness. It is converted to a full-fledged programme for easy installation and execution in windows platform.

The programme works as follows:

- **Step 1:** A screen will appear to the person that instructs how to operate the system. And in second step he has to fiil-up some personal documents.
- **Step 2:** First image comes to the person. There are two figures, one is foreground figure and another is background figure. The person has to identify the foreground figure (*see* Fig. 21.3).
- **Step 3:** If he can identify '8' from the previous image, one identical image with different foreground and background colour will appear to him. Again if he identify '8' as previous,

another identical image come for the another type of colour-blindness. If again he can identify the number '8', a report is generated that shows that he is not colour-blind.

- **Step 4:** Suppose he identifies the foreground figure as '0' in Step 2, then an image appears to him to tell what to do in the next step.
- **Step 5:** After reading the message, which appears to him, he presses the 'OK' button. Then the 'No' button is to be clicked repeatedly up to when he can identify the number '8' from the foreground image. Then when he can identify the number '8' properly, the 'Yes' button is to be clicked (*see* Fig. 21.4).
- **Step 6:** After reading the message that appears to him, he presses the 'OK' button. Now again the same process is to be done for the second half of the wavelength. When he can identify the number '8' the 'Yes' button is to be pressed as follows (*see* Fig. 21.5).
- **Step 7:** Finally the test report appears that shows the final range of colour-blindness (*see* Fig. 21.6).

6. Experimental Results and Conclusions

This programme was tested on about 500 people and out of them we have tested on 20 people who have colour vision problem to some extent. We have got a satisfactory result using our programme. Our programme tells two things, one is the man is colour-blind or not and if he is colour-blind then at what range of wavelength he is colour-blind and also what type of colour-blindness he has. We have also consulted doctors to validate the result obtained by our programme. We have not only tested the result but also the band in which he is colour-blind.

There are so many tests on colour blindness that can tell weather a person is colour-blind or not but we could not find any system that can reveal the band of region where the person is colour-blind. This project is built for identification the band of region where a colour-blind people cannot identify a particular portion of colour. This is an automatic system where every man can test himself whether he is colour-blind or not and if he is colour-blind than he can know in which band of colour he is colour-blind. We have tested on 500 people and have got encouraging results.

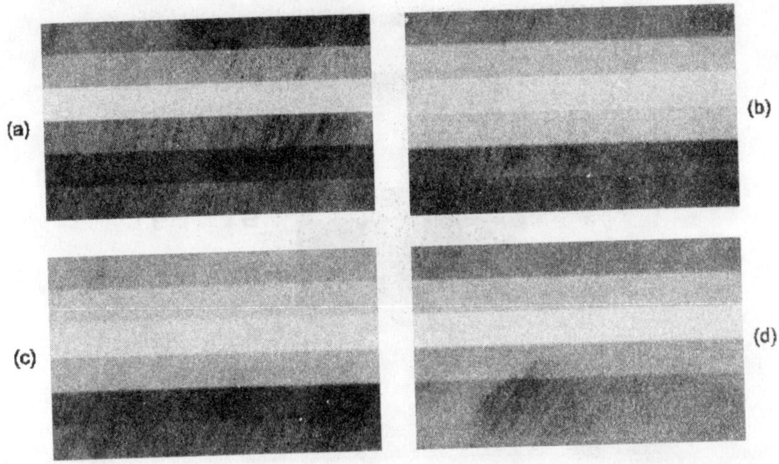

Fig. 21.1: The Colours of the Rainbow as Viewed by a Person with (a) Normal Vision, (b) Protanopia, (c) Deuteranopia, and (d) Tritanopia Colour Blindness [http://www.colormatters.com/v_colorblind.html].

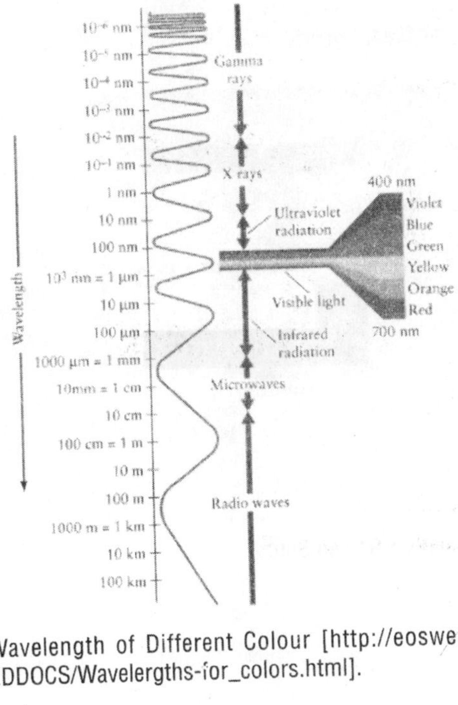

Fig. 21.2: Wavelength of Different Colour [http://eosweb.larc.nasa.gov/EDDOCS/Wavelergths-for_colors.html].

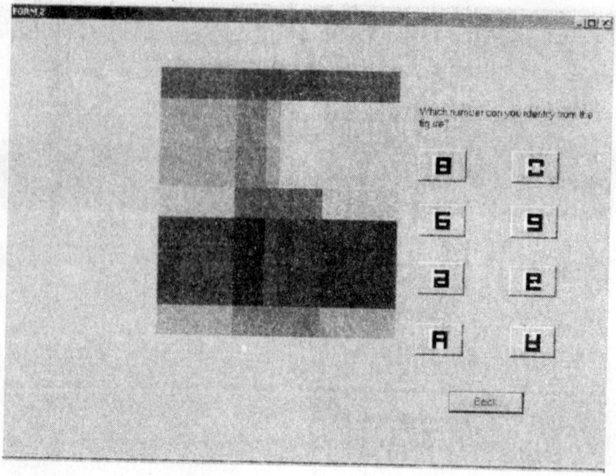

Fig. 21.3: First Screen Shot

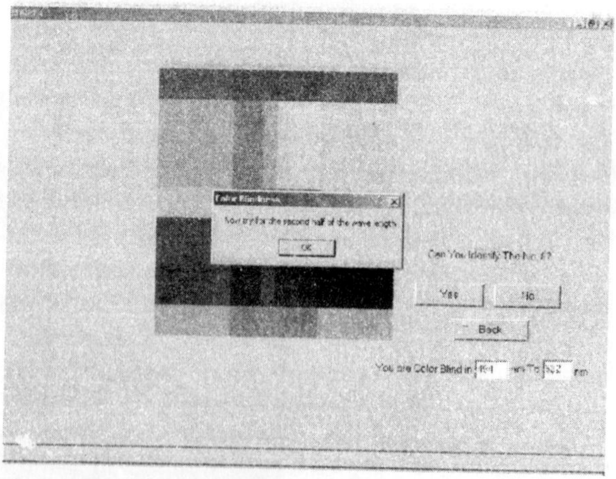

Fig. 21.4: Intermediate Screen Shot

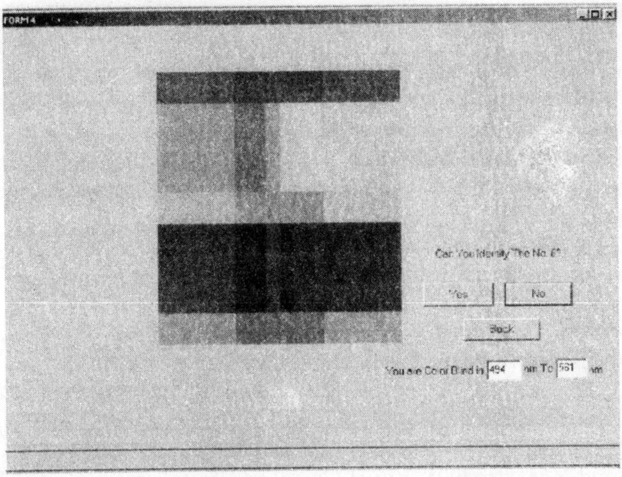

Fig. 21.5: Intermediate Screen Shot

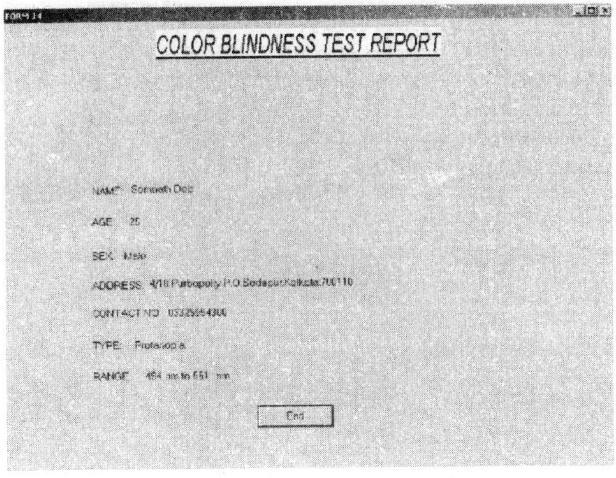

Fig. 21.6: Final Report of Colour-blindness

References

Biernson, G. and A.W. Snyder 1968. A Model of Vision Employing Optical Mode Patterns for Colour Discrimination, *IEEE Systems Science and Cybernetics*, 4 (2):173-181.

Kim, Y.K. with K. Kim and W.X. Yang 2007. Real Time Traffic Light Recognition System for Colour Vision Deficiencies, *Proc. International Conference on Intelligent Robots and Systems*: 333-338.

Kovalev, V.A. 2004. *Towards Image Retrieval for Eight Per cent of Colour-Blind Men,* Proceedings of the Pattern Recognition, 17th International Conference on (ICPR'04) Volume 22: 943-946.

Liu, S. with W. Ma, D. Schalow and K. Spruill 2004. Improving Web Access for Visually Impaired Users, *IEEE Computer Society* 28-33.

Martin, C.E. with J.G. Keller, S.K. Rogers and M. Kabrisky 2000. Colour-Blindness and a Colour Human Visual System Model, *IEEE Systems, Man and Cybernetics, Part A: Systems and Human*, 30 (4): 494-500.

Yang, S. and Y.M. Ro 2003. Visual Contents Adaptation for Colour Vision Deficiency, *Proc. International Conference on Image Processing*, 1: 453-456.

Electronic Document, *http://colorvisiontesting.com/color2.htm*, Accessed February 1, 2010.

Electronic Document, *http://eosweb.larc.nasa.gov/EDDOCS/Wavelengths_for_Colors.html*, Accessed February 1, 2010.

Electronic Document, http:*//www.colormatters.com/v_colorblind.html*, Accessed February 1, 2010.

Electronic Document, *http://www.copresco.com/links/colblind.htm*, Accessed February 1, 2010.

Electronic Document, *http://www.stlukeseye.com/Conditions/ColorBlindness.html*, Accessed February 1, 2010.

Electronic Document, *http://www.toledo-bend.com/colorblind/aboutcb.asp#frustrations*, Accessed February 1, 2010.

Index